Imaging Informatics for Healthcare Professionals

Series Editors

Peter M. A. van Ooijen
Groningen, The Netherlands

Erik R. Ranschaert
Tilburg, The Netherlands

Annalisa Trianni
Udine, Italy

The series Imaging Informatics for Healthcare Professionals is the ideal starting point for physicians and residents and students in radiology and nuclear medicine who wish to learn the basics in different areas of medical imaging informatics. Each volume is a short pocket-sized book that is designed for easy learning and reference.

The scope of the series is based on the Medical Imaging Informatics subsections of the European Society of Radiology (ESR) European Training Curriculum, as proposed by ESR and the European Society of Medical Imaging Informatics (EuSoMII). The series, which is endorsed by EuSoMII, will cover the curricula for Undergraduate Radiological Education and for the level I and II training programmes. The curriculum for the level III training programme will be covered at a later date. It will offer frequent updates as and when new topics arise.

More information about this series at http://link.springer.com/series/16323

Mansoor Fatehi
Daniel Pinto dos Santos
Editors

Structured Reporting in Radiology

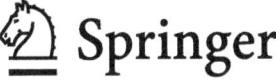 Springer

Editors
Mansoor Fatehi
Biobank
National Brain Mapping
Laboratory
Tehran, Iran

Daniel Pinto dos Santos
Department of Radiology
University Hospital Cologne
Cologne, Germany

ISSN 2662-1541   ISSN 2662-155X   (electronic)
Imaging Informatics for Healthcare Professionals
ISBN 978-3-030-91348-9   ISBN 978-3-030-91349-6   (eBook)
https://doi.org/10.1007/978-3-030-91349-6

This Springer imprint is published by the registered company Springer Nature
Switzerland AG
The registered company address is: Gewerbestrasse 11, 6330 Cham, Switzerland

Preface

Radiology reporting can be defined as the art of converting visually perceptible information into communicable literal documents. The majority of health administrators considers the radiology report as the PRODUCT of radiology department.

Tremendous advancements have taken place in radiology over the past few decades including improvements to a wide range of modalities as well as digital image management from acquisition to advanced visualization. The reporting component of radiology practice has been less affected by such renovations although this component too is now digitalized. Digital transformation has enhanced radiology report management mostly through word processing and voice recognition. But there is a lot to be added to this critical component of the practice, particularly applying digital tools to manage the knowledge delivered within the report both in terms of content and format.

The growing desire for minable medical data in the recent decade has further highlighted the importance of structured reporting because it paves the road for predefined data entry in radiology interpretation which is obviously superior to any retrospective language processing of free text reports. The addition of structured report to daily radiology practice could link busy clinical workflows to research-ready data collection.

Despite rather extensive discussions about structured reporting in radiology, still very little real examples of clinical adoption are evident. Structured reporting (SR) has gone through quite some development stages in the past decades. At the beginning, SR fans tried to convince the so-called regular radiology reporters about advantages of this new method. There are still papers published mainly aiming to highlight benefits of a structured over conventional free text reports. Currently, structured reporting is a well-known subject in medical community, and people are mostly accepting the superiority of this method over others and awareness about SR is sufficiently high.

But in real practice, it has been extremely difficult to merge this method into day-to-day radiology profession. There are multiple challenges from clinical to technical aspects: the depth of structure, flexibility of detailed modules, standard lexicon, interoperability, integration with medical records, back-end issues including database structure and retrieval, DICOM-SR, data representation and report formatting, multimedia attachments and correlations, and so on. For these reasons, not only the end users of structured reporting methods but also the industry partners who are expected to provide practically reliable tools are still looking forward to a better clarified situation.

This book as a part of a larger book series by EuSoMII aims to cover the most important imaging informatics subjects and to address challenges of structured reporting from an interdisciplinary point of view. The book is aimed to cover a diverse audience from clinical users, particularly radiologists, to technical users, namely developers and vendors, as well as researchers who are interested in further expansion of this technology.

Tehran, Iran   Mansoor Fatehi
Cologne, Germany   Daniel Pinto dos Santos

Contents

Language and Radiological Reporting

1

Adrian Brady

Contents

A. Brady (✉)
Radiology Department, Mercy University Hospital, Cork & University College Cork, Cork, Ireland

© European Society of Medical Imaging Informatics (EuSoMII) 2022
M. Fatehi, D. Pinto dos Santos (eds.), *Structured Reporting in Radiology*, Imaging Informatics for Healthcare Professionals, https://doi.org/10.1007/978-3-030-91349-6_1

1

1.1   Introduction

Among characteristics differentiating (most) primates from other mammals are large brains and opposable thumbs (a key requirement for interventional radiologists) [1]. Within the primate order, humans are the only species known to have evolved the ability to communicate using sophisticated spoken language, thought to have arisen 60,000–100,000 years ago [2]. This skill has allowed us develop, enunciate and share complex information and thoughts, including abstract concepts, and has undoubtedly been a major factor in human technological and societal development. However, in some ways, we have been too good in developing language; the Ethnologue website currently lists 7117 recognised spoken languages [3]. The language in which this chapter is being written, English, ranks third by numbers of first-language speakers, after Mandarin Chinese and Spanish [4].

In 1887, Ludwig Zamenhoff, a Polish ophthalmologist, created Esperanto, intended to be a universal second language, designed to promote world peace and international understanding [5]. Although up to 100,000 active users exist around the globe, only about 1000 are native speakers. Its penetration into the world of radiology as a universal communication tool extends only to the use of the name Esperanto for the European Society of Radiology's clinical audit tool [6], the name chosen to reflect the universal applicability of the ESR's clinical audit tool [7].

The children's game known as "telephone" in the United States is called "broken telephone" in many other countries and languages. In Britain, it's called "Chinese whispers", and in the past also "Russian scandal". In France, it's known as "téléphone arabe" (Arabic telephone). The variety of associations with peoples (and presumably languages) other than their own gives an interesting clue as to the game's nature: the first player whispers a message to the second, who in turn whispers the message to the third, and so on through all players. In the end, the message understood by the last player is compared to that whispered by the first. The fun lies in hearing how garbled the original message has become through multiple re-tellings [8]. Sadly, much human communication suffers from the misunderstandings that underpin this game. This is no less true for radiology reporting, which depends for its power on the clear communication of unambiguous information [9]. Believing that our role as radiologists is to make correct diagnoses from imaging data only partly identifies what we should do; communicating our findings and conclusions effectively and clearly is at least as important as the primary interpretation [9]. Radiology reports represent the essential work product of the diagnostic radiologist. Generating those reports can be described as "the art of applying scientific knowledge and understanding to a palette of greys, trying to winnow the relevant and important from the insignificant, seeking to ensure the word-picture we create coheres to a clear and accurate whole, and aiming to be careful advisors regarding appropriate next steps" [10].

From its beginning, radiology as a specialty has understood that radiology reporting should follow a standardised format and language: in 1899, Dr. Preston Hickey, a Michigan radiologist, advocated that reporting of radiographs should follow a standardised format and language [11, 12]. In 1923, Charles Enfield, a Kentucky radiologist, wrote in the Journal of the American Medical Association that a radiology report that does not state what the findings mean "tells much, yet almost nothing" [13]. Until very recently, most publications concerning radiology reporting focused on style and careful word usage. In 1998, Armas summarised the qualities of a good report as the six Cs:

1. Clear
2. Correct
3. Confidence level (which should be indicated)
4. Concise
5. Complete
6. Consistent

all of which come together as the seventh "C": communication [14].

Many authors have suggested ways of structuring and using language in traditional textual reports to minimise ambiguity and optimise clarity, ranging from advice to avoid ambiguous words and phrases ("no evidence of …" [15], "apparent, appears, possible, borderline, doubtful, suspected, indeterminate…suggested, suspected, suspicious for, vague, equivocal, no definite, no gross, no obvious" [16]), eschewing "normal imposters" ("unremarkable, essentially normal, relatively normal, no radiographically visible signs of disease, no significant abnormalities" [13]), resisting the temptation to avoid committing oneself ("clinical correlation recommended" [13]), etc. [9]. As structured reporting becomes increasingly the norm, many of these imprecise word uses are of decreasing relevance.

Over the past 50 years, there have been a series of organised initiatives and developments, initially aimed at standardising the meaning and usage of terms within radiology reports, evolving through standardising the form in which these terms are used and presented to readers, to current systems which structure radiology reports in such a manner that they can be machine-read and interrogated for terms and outcomes facilitating data mining, radiomics and research. For a given examination and clinical context, structured reports should list the same major elements in the same order, regardless of author [13]. The remainder of this chapter will focus not so much on the actual structure of reports, but on this evolution of the language used within reports, and available methods of ensuring this is reproducible and standard, regardless of the reporting radiologist and/or institution.

1.2   Terminologies and Ontologies

Before we review the history of available reporting language systems, it is important to understand a few overall terms. Terminologies refer to sets of terms that have agreed and clearly-defined meanings in the context within which they are used. Beyond encouraging radiologists to report the same abnormality in the same way, the advantages of using defined and controlled terminologies for radiology reporting include allowing computer applications recognise that multiple synonymous terms refer to the same entity, facilitating data mining and query by ensuring that radiological information is included in reports in a standard manner and helping developers create new radiology applications, including structured reporting, coded radiology teaching files and decision support [17]. Radiologists understand that using standard report terms and structures will improve their clarity and reduce individual variability [17].

When using structured reporting, two key elements must be included: consistent organisation and controlled terminology. The terminology must include imaging procedures and techniques, clinical information, diseases and diagnoses etc.

"Ontology" is a term that means more than just a terminology; it includes terms, their attributes and inter-relationships, and is not confined to a specific storage syntax. Thus, while a terminology may be an ontology, not all ontologies are terminologies (their characteristics and uses may go beyond the strict limits of a terminology). A further advantage of ontologies is that they are both readable by humans and processable by computers [17].

1.3   Standard Terminologies

In 1969, eight radiologists met to form a new society to study chest disease primarily through chest radiology, naming themselves the Fleischner Society (in memory of the recently deceased Austrian–American radiologist, Dr. Felix Flesichner). One of the major achievements of the society has been the periodic publication of white papers (formal statements), which have become accepted as standards in chest imaging [18]. In 1984, the Society published the first "Glossary of terms for thoracic radiology" [19], followed by the "Glossary of terms for CT of the lungs" in 1996 [20]. Both of these were superseded by the "Glossary of terms for thoracic imaging" in 2008 [21]. The aim of these publications was to define terms used in thoracic radiology clearly and to encourage standardisation of the usage of these terms. In their publication of the first iteration of this glossary, the Society Nomenclature Committee wrote that they "attempted to indicate whether specific terms are truly descriptors or are, in fact, diagnostic conclusions; and if the latter, whether or not they can appropriately be based solely on radiographic evidence" [19]. This endeavour has been magnificently successful in forming the thought processes of thoracic radiologists the world over, ensuring that, as far as is possible, the same terms are used in the same way to mean the same thing. An example is the encouragement to use the preferred term "consolidation" rather than less-specific synonyms such as "airspace opacity", "parenchymal opacification" or "infiltrate".

In 2001, the North American Spine Society, the American Society of Spine Radiology and the American Society of Neuroradiology published recommendations for nomenclature and classification of lumbar disc pathology [22], which aimed to achieve a similar standardisation of the use of terminology in this specific area of radiology. Version 2 of these recommendations, published in 2014 [23], updated the terminology, again with the aim of ensuring accurate and consistent use of standard terms.

Also in 2001, Atkinson et al. described a system of reporting terminology for radiographic and clinical features of brain arteriovenous malformations [24].

In 2002, an international interdisciplinary committee published recommended terminology to be used with respect to lower limb veins; a further update was published in 2005 [25].

Probably the best-known system of standardisation of reporting language derives from the Breast Imaging Reporting and Data System (BI-RADS), developed by the American College of Radiology (ACR). With increasing utilisation of mammography in the 1980s, the lack of standardisation of practices was recognised as a problem. The American Medical Association (AMA) stated that "mammography reports too often contained unintelligible descriptions and ambiguous recommendations" [26]. In 1986, the ACR convened a committee to develop a voluntary mammography accreditation program, out of which grew a separate committee tasked with drafting guidelines on mammography reporting and management (BI-RADS). The first version of the guidelines was published in 1993 and included recommendations for the conduct of mammography, an overall structure for mammography reports, final assessment categories with management recommendations and a mammography lexicon [26, 27]. The terms within the BI-RADS lexicon were defined precisely, to eliminate ambiguity, and were chosen to be evidence-based and predictive, to ensure clear and accurate communication of mammography findings [26]. Furthermore, the committee recommended that reports be summarised by choosing only one of a set of standardised final assessment categories at the end of a report, each of which included a matched, standardised management recommendation (Category 0—need additional imaging evaluation and/or prior mammograms for comparison; Category 1—negative; Category 2—benign finding(s); Category 3—probably benign finding, initial short-interval follow-up recommended; Category 4—suspicious abnormality, biopsy should be considered; Category 5—highly suggestive of malignancy, appropriate action should be taken; Category 6—known biopsy-proven malignancy, appropriate action should be taken) [26].

BI-RADS has not remained static since its inception. After first publication in 1993, further editions, modifications and clarifications appeared in 1995, 1998, 2003 and 2007. An Atlas was incorporated in the third edition (1998) to illustrate each descriptor. A breast ultrasound lexicon, BI-RADS-ULTRASOUND, was added in the fourth edition (2003), as were breast MRI descriptors [26]. The fifth and current edition was published in 2013 [28], and has been translated into Spanish, German, Portuguese, Chinese, Japanese and Greek [29]. The standardisation of breast imaging reporting via the BI-RADS system has been of great benefit, aligning the language used by radiologists to clinical categorisation and decision-making, and permitting multi-institutional data collection, data sharing and auditing and comparison [13].

Since the success of BI-RADS, similar approaches have been taken for imaging other organs and body systems. In 2008, the ACR convened a group of expert radiologists to develop a comprehensive system for interpreting and reporting CTs and MRs of the liver in patients at risk of hepatocellular carcinoma (HCC). This led to the official launch in March 2011 of LI-RADS (Liver Imaging Reporting and Data System) [30, 31]. Other ACR-supported similar reporting systems and tools include C-RADS (CT Colonography Reporting and Data System) [32], CAD-RADS (Coronary Artery Disease Reporting and Data System) [33], HI-RADS (Head Injury Imaging Reporting and Data System) [34], Lung-RADS (Lung CT Screening Report and Data

System) [35], NI-RADS (Neck Imaging Reporting and Data System) [36], O-RADS (Ovarian-Adnexal Reporting and Data System) [37], PI-RADS (Prostate Imaging Reporting and Data System) [38] and TI-RADS (Thyroid Imaging Reporting and Data System) [39]. Other academic bodies have also contributed to these standards; for example, in 2012, the European Society of Urogenital Radiology (ESUR) published guidelines for prostate MRI reporting [40].

As the amount of imaging utilisation and medical data availability grew massively from the 1980s, other, more general efforts were made to standardise biomedical terminology. In 1986, the US National Library of Medicine (NLM) designed and constructed the Unified Medical Language System (UMLS) to collect and link controlled vocabularies to facilitate the development of computer systems that could understand, retrieve and classify biomedical literature. Components of UMLS are used by the NLM for its PubMed system [26]. It now incorporates more than 200 biomedical content resources [41].

Systems, such as BI-RADS and other similar systems are largely specifications of best practices for creating reports in specific clinical contexts. They detail the types of information which should be included in a radiology report, and the descriptive terms that should be used, but they don't explicitly describe the model of information to be included in a report, and do not create a specification permitting data interoperability [42]. Development and refinement of multi-modality structured reporting systems, applicable beyond single organs or body systems, required further steps in standardising radiology (and other medical) language meanings, use, and inter-relationships, which have been addressed by some of the following systems.

1.4 LOINC

LOINC (Logical Observation Identifier Names and Codes) is a freely available global standard code system for reporting laboratory and other clinical observations in HL7 messages [43] (HL7 International is a standard-developing organisation that provides standards and framework for the exchange, integration, sharing and retrieval of electronic health information [44]). Its primary role is to provide identifiers and names for observations (i.e. health data represented in a particular way, tests, variables or data elements) [45]. LOINC was developed in 1994 by the Regenstrief Institute (a non-profit medical research organisation associated with Indiana University) in Indianapolis [45] and its initial release in May 1995 contained identifiers and names for over 6000 laboratory test results [43]. By December 1996, LOINC had added about 1500 clinical measurement terms, such as vital signs, ECG measurements etc. [45]. By 2003, LOINC was being used in DICOM ultrasound messages [43] and by 2018, after more than 60 further releases, it had expanded in other domains, including radiology [45]. LOINC clinical observation names are defined in terms of six major and up to four minor axes [43]. It currently contains over 85,000 codes [41].

The LOINC Committee now comprises three major composite committees: Laboratory, Clinical and Radiology. New releases occur twice yearly. LOINC has become widely adopted as a standard for lab and clinical observations in the United States and internationally [45]. It is used by the US Centers for Disease Control (CDC) and Veterans Administration (VA) [43]. Overall, there are more than 60,000 registered users in 170 countries. LOINC has been translated into 18 variants of 12 languages, and more than 30 countries (including Switzerland, Hong Kong, Australia Canada and the German Institute for Standardization {DIN—Deutsche Institut für Normung}) have adopted LOINC as a national standard [43].

Within and among health IT systems, observations are communicated with a structure that has two key structural elements. The first identifies what the observation is (e.g. diastolic blood pressure), and the second carries the result value (e.g. 80 mm Hg). When used together, these two elements carry an instance of a specific test result for a given pt. A common pairing is to use LOINC as the standard code for the observation and SNOMED CT (see subsequently) as the standard code for the observation value [45]. If we consider a test observation as a question and observation values as the answers, LOINC provides codes for the questions, and other systems, e.g. SNOMED CT, provide codes for the answers [43].

The Regenstrief Institute and the RSNA have unified the RadLex Playbook (see subsequently) and LOINC radiology terms to produce a single comprehensive system for naming and coding radiology examinations, constructed using RadLex terms, with a shared governance [41].

1.5   SNOMED CT

In 1965, the College of American Pathologists (CAP) developed the Structured Nomenclature of Pathology (SNOP), containing about 15,000 distinct medical objects, processes and concepts [44, 45]. Around the same time, under the auspices of the British National Health Service (NHS), Dr. James Read developed the Read codes, which evolved into Clinical terms Version 3 (CTV-3). In 2002, CTV-3 and SNOMED Reference Terminology (SNOMED RT, a further evolution of SNOP) combined to create SNOMED CT (SNOMED Clinical Terms), a joint development project of the NHS and CAP [44]. The first SNOMED CT release in Jan 2003 contained 278,000 active concepts. The January 2018 release of SNOMED CT had 341,000 concepts, 1,062,000 active relationships and 1,156,000 active descriptions [45], enlarged in the January 31, 2020 release of the SNOMED CT International Edition to 352,567 concepts, comprising diagnoses, clinical findings, surgical, therapeutic and diagnostic procedures, observables, concepts representing body structures, organisms, substances, pharmaceutical products, physical objects, physical specimens, forces etc. [46]. Updated versions are released twice a year; 22% of the contained concepts are disorders, 17% procedures, 11% body structures, 10% clinical findings other than disorders and 10% organisms [45].

SNOMED CT contains only 4000 textual definitions of concepts. Rather, its descriptions are labels that describe concepts. Its design criterion is to keep concept expressions simple enough to be broadly usable by clinicians while maintaining a faithful representation of the meaning of a concept [45].

The core component types within SNOMED CT are concepts, descriptions and relationships. Every concept within SNOMED CT represents a unique clinical meaning, referenced using a unique, numeric and machine-readable SNOMED CT identifier, which provides an unambiguous unique reference to each concept and does not have any ascribed human interpretable meaning. Two types of descriptions are used to represent every concept, the Fully Specified Name (FSN) and Synonyms. The FSN represents a unique, unambiguous description of a concept's meaning (particularly useful when different concepts are referred to by the same commonly used word or phrase). Each concept can have only one FSN in any language or dialect. A synonym represents a term that can be used to display or select a concept (which may have several synonyms), allowing users of SNOMED CT to use the terms they prefer to refer to a specific clinical meaning. A relationship represents an association between two concepts. Relationships are used to logically define the meaning of a concept in a way that can be processed by a computer. A third concept, called a relationship type (or attribute), is used to represent the meaning of the association between the source and destination concepts [46].

SNOMED CT ownership was transferred to the newly formed not-for-profit International Health Terminology Development Standards Organisation (IHTDSO) in 2007, subsequently renamed SNOMED International. Initially, the IHTDSO had nine member countries, with a combined population of about 500 million: United States, United Kingdom, Canada, Australia and New Zealand (official language English) and others with other languages (Netherlands, Sweden, Denmark, Lithuania). As of May 2018, the organisation covers 32 countries with a combined population of over two billion, with a broad range of languages. Partial or full translations of SNOMED CT have been developed in Danish, Dutch, French, Spanish and Swedish [45].

SNOMED CT is increasingly engaged in collaboration and harmonisation with other relevant standards; this involves mapping of SNOMED CT terms with WHO classifications (e.g. the WHO International Classification of Diseases ICD-10, the International Classification for Nursing Practice ICNP and

LOINC {a cooperation agreement was reached in 2013 between the Regenstrief Institute, representing LOINC, and SNOMED International}) [45, 46].

SNOMED CT has other domain-specific collaborations, with Orphanet for harmonisation of content with ORDO (Orphanet ontology of rare diseases), and with the Global Medical Device Nomenclature Agency (GMDNA) for medical device terminology [45].

National extensions to SNOMED CT are also possible for member countries of SNOMED International; typically these contain concepts important in a given country, but not in scope for international releases of SNOMED CT [45].

LOINC, SNOMED CT and RxNorm (a standard drug ontology from the United States) have been selected as the terminological backbone of the Observational Medical Outcomes Partnership (OMOP) common data model (CDM) used for clinical data warehouses internationally by OHDSI (Observational Health Data Sciences and Informatics collective) [45]. SNOMED, HL7 and LOINC have been endorsed by the American Veterinary Medical Association as the official informatics standards in veterinary medicine in the United States [44].

The DICOM (Digital Imaging and Communications in Medicine—the international standards to transmit, store, retrieve, print, process and display medical imaging information [47]) Standards Committee has chosen SNOMED CT as its primary source of terminology and has created the DICOM Controlled Terminology resource to create terms when existing resources do not contain needed terms [48]. In March 2016, the IHTDSO and DICOM signed a 5-year SNOMED CT licensing agreement, clarifying the use of an agreed set of more than 7000 SNOMED CT codes and descriptions in DICOM standards [46].

1.6 FMA

The Foundational Model of Anatomy (FMA) is a reference ontology of human anatomy, from the macromolecular to the organism scale, developed at the University of Washington in Seattle. It contains approx. 75,000 anatomic concepts and >2.1 million relationships [41].

1.7   ACR Index and RadLex

The American College of Radiology (ACR) Index for Radiological Diagnoses was first published in 1955, with subsequent editions in 1961,1986 and 1992 [49] and remained the standard system for classifying radiology teaching cases for decades. It consisted of a digital code containing up to nine digits. The first 2–4 digits, prior to a decimal point, defined the anatomical part described; the digits (2–5) after the decimal represented the pathological diagnosis. The more digits in the identifier, the more specific was the description [50]. In 1999, the ACR released the Index in digital format on CD-ROM. In 1994, a web-based version was developed. A poster-sized version of the Index was formerly a common sight on radiologists' office walls; indeed, the author still possesses a cabinet containing an almost entirely redundant collection of about 1200 meticulously indexed (following the ACR system) library of cut-film teaching cases, accumulated from the late 1980s on, and now almost never used.

Although the ACR index was of great value in classifying case diagnoses, the amount of information which could be coded was quite limited and largely confined to diagnoses or anatomical observations. It contained only a few thousand unique terms. Furthermore, the fixed relationship between digital codes and concepts made it difficult to retire or add terms without changing the codes of other nearby concepts. In summary, the ACR index was designed for human memory and information processing ability, and in the computer age, this became its main deficiency [50].

About 20 years ago, the Radiological Society of North America (RSNA) developed the Medical Imaging Resource Center (MIRC), a set of tools enabling users to connect and share teaching files over the internet, evolving into a server hosting teaching cases. This project quickly encountered the problem that, at the time, no medical terminological system was available to adequately meet the needs of online radiology indexing, largely because of the lack of any complete set of imaging terms [50]. Therefore, in spring 2003, 12 radiologists convened to consider a first draft of thoracic anatomy terms as the beginning of the RSNA RadLex ("lexicon for uniform indexing and retrieval of radiology information resources" [48]) project. Following this successful pilot, the development of RadLex terminology began in earnest in 2005, designed to create a single source for medical imaging terminology. Approximately 12,000 terms were released publicly in conjunction with the RSNA meeting in 2007 [13]. The initial principal goal was to allow annotation, indexing and retrieval of information from MIRC. The ACR contributed the ACR Index to RadLex, and an arrangement was made with the College of American Pathologists to use a subset of SNOMED CT terms as a starting point for the RadLex lexicon [50].

Very early in its evolution, RadLex added substantially to the anatomical and pathological codes of the ACR Index, incorporating codes for devices, procedures and imaging techniques, the perceptual and analytical difficulty of the interpretation and the diagnostic quality of the images [50]. RadLex was designed to be continuously supplemented and updated with incorporation of new concepts, including harmonisation with other popular medical vocabularies and sets of terms, such as SNOMED-CT, ICD10, CPT (Current Procedural Terminology, from the American Medical Association), BrainInfo (a project of the National Primate Research Centre of the University of Washington [51]) and the ACR Index [50].

RadLex is an ontology organised fundamentally along a type hierarchy, also called the "Is-A" hierarchy. This defines parent (class) and child (subclass) relationships, where a given subclass is a kind or type of its parent (e.g. the left lung is a subclass of the concept "lung"). The left upper lobe is not a subclass of "left lung", but is part of the anatomical left lung and is encoded using a "Has-Part" relationship. Thus, the left upper lobe is a subclass of "upper lobe of lung", which is in turn a subclass of "lobe of lung" [41].

RadLex, likes other terminologies, consists of terms and attributes of terms. By 2018, it contained over 45,000 concepts. RadLex assigns a unique code (RadLex Identifier or RID) and a preferred name to each of these concepts. Synonyms (alternate ways of naming the preferred terms) or translations may also be attached to each concept [17, 41].

The RadLex ontology aims to provide a comprehensive resource for imaging-related terms, incl. imaging technologies, imaging findings, anatomy and pathology. It has not been without its difficulties. Its original flat file format was relatively friendly to human users, but cumbersome for structural analysis and detection of omissions, duplications and inconsistency ("curation" of the terminology). Also, because RadLex changes over time, difficulties were encountered updating all client applications and disseminating new versions when changes were released [17].

The RadLex Playbook is a catalogue of all studies that can be performed in a radiology dept. (all the "plays" that can be called in a radiology dept.); the sporting metaphor was first suggested by Betsy Humphries of the National Library of Medicine. Early versions of the Playbook were bloated by very many codes that essentially described the same or very similar procedures. It has subsequently been revised to a "Core Playbook", with removal of many duplications [13]. The RadLex Playbook was translated into German by the Deutsche Röntgengesellschaft (DRG) in 2017 and is currently being translated into Portuguese [52].

A further refinement of the various systems of nomenclature described here is the concept of Common Data Elements (CDEs), which will be further detailed in Chap. 7. In essence, CDEs represent predefined questions and the set of allowable answers to each question. They can be thought of as data elements that can be collected and stored uniformly across studies and institutions, defined in a dictionary which specifies the item's name, data type (e.g. text or numerical), allowable values and other attributes (including information telling applications systems how to use them) [42]. CDEs can be indexed according to controlled terms from vocabularies such as LOINC, SNOMED-CT and RadLex, and further refine RadLex by ensuring consistent standardised language and organisation in radiology reports, with uniform data capture, which in turn permits multi-institutional or population-based radiology research [42]. Thus, structured reports ordered in a consistent manner and using standardised language, with codable CDEs forming the basis of the report, are required and ideal for data mining [53] and radiomics, and also allow the integration of tools to assist radiologists, such as automatic TNM classification [48].

1.8   Summary

From its earliest days, it was recognised that radiology reports should use clear, unambiguous language, in a manner that made the meaning of reports immediately understandable to referrers. Nonetheless, radiology reporting remained a text-based exercise, highly dependent for its quality and clarity on the individual word choices, styles and efforts of radiologists. From the 1980s onwards, increasing attention has been paid to the need to standardise reporting language, to avoid ambiguity and misinterpretation. Attention then became directed at actual report structures, defining precisely how standardised language should be presented. With the advent of medical informatics, these two elements (language and structure) are being combined and integrated, increasingly facilitating comparison and understanding of reports, regardless of where or by whom they are initially generated. The development of terminologies and ontologies outlined in this chapter has advanced this standardisation, and the integration of systems from different sources into specialty-specific tools, such as RadLex, shows the future of radiology reports, instantly transferable among institutions and countries, and searchable (regardless of source) for data and elements. The power of multi-centre radiology research will be greatly enhanced by the use of standardised radiology report language and structures, heralding a new era of patient and population benefit that goes far beyond traditional observation and diagnosis.

References

1. Wikipedia: Primate. https://en.wikipedia.org/wiki/Primate. Accessed 6 May 2020.
2. Wikipedia: Language. https://en.wikipedia.org/wiki/Language#Distinctive_features_of_human_language. Accessed 6 May 2020.
3. Ethnologue: Languages of the world. https://www.ethnologue.com/about. Accessed 6 May 2020.
4. Wikipedia: List of languages by number of native speakers. https://en.wikipedia.org/wiki/List_of_languages_by_number_of_native_speakers. Accessed 6 May 2020.

5. Wikipedia: Esperanto. https://en.wikipedia.org/wiki/Esperanto. Accessed 6 May 2020.
6. European Society of Radiology: The Esperanto booklet. https://www.myesr.org/quality-safety/clinical-audit. Accessed 6 May 2020.
7. European Society of Radiology (ESR). The ESR Audit Tool (Esperanto): genesis, contents & pilot. Insights Imaging. 2018;9:899–903. https://doi.org/10.1007/s13244-018-0651-0.
8. Wikipedia: Chinese whispers. https://en.wikipedia.org/wiki/Chinese_whispers. Accessed 6 May 2020.
9. Brady AP. Radiology reporting—from Hemingway to HAL? Insights Imaging. 2018;9:237–46. https://doi.org/10.1007/s13244-018-0596-.
10. Brady AP. Error and discrepancy in radiology—inevitable or avoidable? Insights Imaging. 2017;8:171–82. https://doi.org/10.1007/s13244-016-0534-1.
11. Wallis A, McCoubrie P. The radiology report—are we getting the message across? Clin Radiol. 2011;66:1015–22.
12. Murray J. The early formative years in Irish Radiology. In: Carr JC, editor. A century of medical radiation in ireland—an anthology. Dublin: Anniversary Press; 1995. p. 9.
13. Langlotz CP. The radiology report. Stanford, CA: Langlotz; 2015. ISBN 978-1515174080.
14. Armas RR. Letter: qualities of a good radiology report. AJR. 1998;170:1110.
15. Friedman PJ. Radiologic reporting: structure. AJR. 1983;140:171–2.
16. Hall FM. Language of the radiology report; Primer for residents and wayward radiologists. AJR. 2000;175:1239–42.
17. Rubin DL. Creating and curating a terminology for radiology: ontology modeling and analysis. J Digit Imaging. 2008;21(4):355–62.
18. Janower ML. A brief history of the Fleischner Society. J Thorac Imaging. 2010;25:27–8. https://doi.org/10.1097/RTI.0b013e3181cc4cee.
19. Tuddenham WJ. Glossary of terms for thoracic radiology: recommendations of the Nomenclature Committee of the Fleischner Society. AJR Am J Roentgenol. 1984;143:509–17. https://doi.org/10.2214/ajr.143.3.509.
20. Austin JH, Müller NL, Friedman PJ, et al. Glossary of terms for CT of the lungs: recommendations of the Nomenclature Committee of the Fleischner Society. Radiology. 1996;200:327–31.
21. Hansell DM, Bankier AA, MacMahon H, et al. Fleischner Society: glossary of terms for thoracic imaging. Radiology. 2008;246:697–722. https://doi.org/10.1148/radiol.2462070712.
22. Fardon DF, Milette PC. Nomenclature and classification of lumbar disc pathology: recommendations of the combined task forces of the North American Spine Society, the American Society of Spine Radiology and the American Society of Neuroradiology. Spine. 2001;26:E93–113.
23. Fardon DF, Williams AL, Dohring EJ, Murtagh FR, Gabriel Rothman SL, Sze GK. Lumbar disc nomenclature: version 2.0: recommendations of the

combined task forces of the North American Spine Society, the American Society of Spine Radiology and the American Society of Neuroradiology. Spine J Off J North Am Spine Soc. 2014;14:2525–45.

24. Atkinson RP, et al. Reporting terminology for brain arteriovenous malformation clinical and radiographic features for use in clinical trials. Stroke. 2001;32:1430–42.

25. Caggiati A, et al. Nomenclature of the veins of the lower limbs: an international; interdisciplinary consensus statement. J Vasc Surg. 2002;36:416–22.

26. Burnside ES, Sickles EA, Bassett LW, Rublin DL, Lee CH, Ikeda DM, Mendelson EB, Wilcox PA, Butler PF, D'Orsi CJ. The ACR BI-RADS experience: learning from history. J Am Coll Radiol. 2009;6:851–60. https://doi.org/10.1016/j.jacr.2009.07.023.

27. American College of Radiology. ACR practice guideline for the performance of screening and diagnostic mammography. In: Practice guidelines and technical standards. Reston, VA: American College of Radiology; 2008. p. 525–34.

28. D'Orsi CJ, Sickles EA, Mendelson EB, Morris EA, et al. ACR BI-RADS® Atlas, breast imaging reporting and data system. Reston, VA: American College of Radiology; 2013.

29. American College of Radiology: The American College of Radiology BI-RADS Atlas 5th Edition: Frequently asked questions. https://www.acr.org/-/media/ACR/Files/RADS/BI-RADS/BIRADSFAQ.pdf. Accessed 9 June 2020.

30. Mitchell DG, Bruix J, Sherman M, Sirlin CB. LI-RADS (Liver Imaging Reporting and Data System): summary, discussion and consensus of the LI_RADS management working group and future directions. Hepatology. 2015;61:1056–65.

31. American College of Radiology: Liver Reporting and Data System (LI-RADS). https://www.acr.org/Clinical-Resources/Reporting-and-Data-Systems/LI-RADS. Accessed 9 June 2020.

32. American College of Radiology: CT Colonography Reporting and Data System (C-RADS). https://www.acr.org/Clinical-Resources/Reporting-and-Data-Systems/C-Rads. Accessed 18 June 2020.

33. American College of Radiology: Coronary Artery Disease Reporting and Data System. https://www.acr.org/Clinical-Resources/Reporting-and-Data-Systems/Cad-Rads. Accessed 9 June 2020.

34. American College of Radiology: Head Injury Imaging Reporting and Data System (HI-RADS). https://www.acr.org/Clinical-Resources/Reporting-and-Data-Systems/HI-RADS. Accessed 9 June 2020.

35. American College of Radiology: Lung Cancer Screening Reporting and Data System (Lung-RADS). https://www.acr.org/Clinical-Resources/Reporting-and-Data-Systems/Lung-Rads. Accessed 9 June 2020.

36. American College of Radiology: Neck Imaging Reporting and Data System (NI-RADS). https://www.acr.org/Clinical-Resources/Reporting-and-Data-Systems/NI-RADs. Accessed 9 June 2020.

37. American College of Radiology: Ovarian-Adnexal Reporting and Data System (O-RADS). https://www.acr.org/Clinical-Resources/Reporting-and-Data-Systems/O-Rads. Accessed 9 June 2020.
38. American College of Radiology: Prostate Imaging Reporting and Data System (PI-RADS). https://www.acr.org/Clinical-Resources/Reporting-and-Data-Systems/PI-RADS. Accessed 9 June 2020.
39. American College of Radiology: Thyroid Imaging Reporting and Data System (TI-RADS). https://www.acr.org/Clinical-Resources/Reporting-and-Data-Systems/TI-RADS. Accessed 9 June 2020.
40. Barentsz JO, et al. Prostate MR guidelines 2012. Eur Radiol. 2012;22:746–57.
41. Wang KC. Standard lexicons, coding systems and ontologies for interoperability and semantic computation in imaging. J Digit Imaging. 2018;31:353–60. https://doi.org/10.1007/s10278-018-0069-8.
42. Rubin DL, Kahn CE. Common data elements in radiology. Radiology. 2017;283:837–44. https://doi.org/10.1148/radiol.2016161553.
43. McDonald CJ, Huff SM, Suico JG, et al. LOINC, a universal standard for identifying laboratory observations: a 5-year update. Clin Chem. 2003;49(4):624–33.
44. Awaysheh A, Wilcke J, Elvinger F, Rees L, Fan W, Zimmerman K. A review of medical terminology standards and structured reporting. J Vet Diagn Investig. 2018;30:17–25. https://doi.org/10.1177/1040638717738276.
45. Bodenreider O, Cornet R, Freeman DJ. Recent developments in clinical terminologies—SNOMED CT, LOINC, and RxNorm. Yearb Med Inform. 2018:129–39. https://doi.org/10.1055/s-0038-1667077.
46. SNOMED International. https://www.snomed.org. Accessed 18 June 2020.
47. DICOM: Digital Imaging and Communication in Medicine. https://www.dicomstandard.org. Accessed 17 June 2020.
48. European Society of Radiology. ESR paper on Structured Reporting in Radiology. Insights Imaging. 2018;9:1–7. https://doi.org/10.1007/s13244-017-0588-8.
49. ACR Index: American College of Radiology. Index for radiological diagnoses. 4th ed. Reston, VA; 1992, ISBN 1-55903-134-4.
50. Langlotz CR. RadLex: a new method for indexing online educational materials. Radiographics. 2006;26:1595–7.
51. National Primate Research Center: BrainInfo. http://braininfo.rprc.washington.edu/copyright.aspx. Accessed 18 June 2020.
52. Radiological Society of North America: RadLex radiology lexicon. https://www.rsna.org/en/practice-tools/data-tools-and-standards/radlex-radiology-lexicon. Accessed 18 June 2020.
53. Bozkurt S, Kahn CE Jr. An open-standards grammar for outline-style radiology report templates. J Digit Imaging. 2012;25:359–64. https://doi.org/10.1007/S10278-012-9456-8.

Standardized Reporting Systems

2

Bijan Bijan, Pavel Gelezhe ⓘ,
Ivan Blokhin ⓘ, Aleksander Nikolaev ⓘ,
and Sergey Morozov ⓘ

Contents

B. Bijan
Department of Radiology, University of California Davis Medical
Center, Sacramento, CA, USA

P. Gelezhe · I. Blokhin · A. Nikolaev · S. Morozov (✉)
Research and Practical Clinical Center of Diagnostics and Telemedicine
Technologies, Department of Health Care of Moscow, Moscow, Russia
e-mail: i.blokhin@npcmr.ru; s.morozov@npcmr.ru

© European Society of Medical Imaging Informatics
(EuSoMII) 2022
M. Fatehi, D. Pinto dos Santos (eds.), *Structured Reporting in
Radiology*, Imaging Informatics for Healthcare Professionals,
https://doi.org/10.1007/978-3-030-91349-6_2

2.1   Introduction

2.1.1   Basic Concepts of Standardized Reporting Systems

Reporting and data systems (RADS) are guidelines for the evaluation and interpretation of imaging studies. Each system is developed by a consensus panel of experts and can be updated periodically to improve diagnostic efficacy. Standardized reports are preferable to both radiologists and referring physicians as they minimize variations in reports and ambiguity in terminology.

Besides, the systematic nature of ACR RADS allows for consistent data collection. These qualities are critical to facilitate result monitoring, as well as to improve acceptance and quality assurance.

2.1.2   Advantages of Standardized Reporting Systems

- Usage of a common lexicon facilitates communication.
- Nonstandard terminology is discouraged, avoiding ambiguities.
- Standardizing the image acquisition technique, with more uniform protocols across the globe.
- Each scoring system corresponds to the degree of suspected disease/condition.
- Offering standard follow-up recommendations for each specific category.
- Providing a checklist to the radiologist, providing uniformity, and avoiding misses.
- Easy to follow reports (easy on eyes).
- Easy access to the information for auditing and data classification (research).
- Easy access to data for epidemiologic purposes.

2.1.3 Disadvantages of Standardized Reporting Systems

- Causes laziness on behalf of radiologists, resulting in embarrassing mistakes.
- Shifting attention to the organ of interest, diverging from other structures included in the study, and potentially missing other important findings.
- The learning curve, although maybe initially steep, plateaus before making another steep curve to the level of expert readers.
- Each structured reporting system is specific to different diseases, and there are inherent structural differences between the systems.
- The critical detail is whether the study readings are intended for screening or diagnosis if scores are given per lesion or patient. The range of numbers is included in the scoring categories.
- There is a relatively long period for SRS updates, possibly leading to suboptimal patient care.
- Some RADS have technical remarks on scanning parameters (PI-RADS, LI-RADS). Others do not (COVID-RADS, CAD-RADS), possibly increasing the discrepancies for future quality assurance and effect analysis.

2.1.4 Clinical Adoption of Standardized Reporting Systems

Clinical applications of ACR RADS vary broadly based on radiologists, institutions, and practice settings. BI-RADS received the most recognition and interest, followed by PI-RADS and LI-RADS, as evidenced by the growing number of publications. Further integration of RADS into clinical society guidelines, as demonstrated by BI-RADS with the American Society of Breast

Surgeons and LI-RADS with the American Liver Association, can increase the use and impact of radiology on clinical care.

2.1.5 Clinical Impact of Standardized Reporting Systems

Structured reporting is paramount for teaching, as each case reflects the probability of clinically significant disease or its severity. SRS may increase data availability for research due to uniform scanning protocols and analysis guidelines. Big data, in turn, leads to the continuous improvement of the RADS. Another output of structured data is validated datasets, which are to be used for training and validation of convolutional neural networks or, in other words, artificial intelligence.

2.1.6 Standardized Reporting Systems and Imaging Informatics

Structured reporting facilitates the adaption to informatics infrastructure of imaging centers. AI application can be much easier with higher accuracy utilizing digested, well-organized imaging data, and reports with the introduction of AI to the clinical practice.

2.1.7 Standardized Reporting Systems and Imaging Management

A sound management strategy needs a sound data collection system. Standard reporting systems can produce a more comprehensive and organized data bank, essential for data categorization and data analysis, which would provide the base for management purposes.

Content:

01:	LI-RADS	Liver/hepatoma
02:	O-RADS	Ovarian lesions
03:	PI-RADS	Prostate cancer
04:	LU-RADS	Lung nodules
05:	BI-RADS	Breast cancer
06:	COVID-RADS	COVID-19 pneumonia
07:	TI-RADS	Thyroid nodules
08:	https://www.acr.org/Clinical-Resources/Reporting-and-Data-Systems/HIRADS	Pending
09:	NI-RADS	Neuro
10:	CAD-RADS	Coronary arterial disease
11:	C-RADS	CT colonography

2.2 LI-RADS

2.2.1 Definition

2.2.1.1 LIRADS: Liver Imaging Reporting and Data System (LI-RADS)

A comprehensive system for standardization of terminology, technique, interpretation, reporting, and data collection of liver imaging.

2.2.2 Applicable Population [1]

LI-RADS classification system should only be applied to the sub-population with significantly increased risk for developing hepatocellular carcinoma (HCC), including

- Cirrhotic liver
- Chronic HBV without cirrhosis
- Current or prior history of HCC (including adult liver transplant candidates, posttransplant recipients)

2.2.3 Avoid Using LI-RADS in the Following Subpopulations

– Without significant risk factor
– Pediatric population (under 18 years of age)
– Cirrhosis due to congenital hepatic fibrosis
– Cirrhosis due to a vascular disorder such as hereditary hemorrhagic telangiectasia, Budd–Chiari syndrome, chronic portal vein occlusion, cardiac congestion, or diffuse nodular regenerative hyperplasia

2.2.4 Technical Remarks [2]

LI-RADS can be applied to the following modalities:

– Multiphase contrast-enhanced CT
– Multiphase contrast-enhanced MR (extracellular contrast agents or hepatobiliary contrast agents)
– Ultrasound

LI-RADS categories should not be used for the following observations:

– Pathologically proven malignancies
– Pathologically proven benign lesions of nonhepatocellular origin such as hemangiomas

LI-RADS has several categories (Table 2.1), with main imaging features (Fig. 2.1) as well as ancillary signs (Table 2.2). Evidence-based statistics and common pitfalls are provided in

Table 2.1 Categories. Which LI-RADS categories are existing?

LR-NC	LR-TIV	LR-1	LR-2	LR-M	LR-3	LR-4	LR-5
Not categorizable (due to image omission or degradation)	Tumor in vein	Definitely benign	Probably benign	Probably or definitely malignant, but not necessarily HCC	Intermediate probability of HCC	Probably HCC (Fig. 2.2)	Definitely HCC

| Non-rim arterial phase enhancement unequivocally greater in whole or in part than liver.

Enhancing part must be higher in attenuation or intensity than liver in arterial phase | Nonperipheral "washout"

Nonperipheral visually assessed temporal reduction in enhancement in whole or in part relative to composite liver tissue from earlier to later phase resulting in hypoenhancement in the extracellular phase | Enhancing capsule

Capsule: peripheral rim of smooth hyperenhancement seen in the portal venous, transitional or delayed phase |

| Threshold growth:
Diameter increase >50% in <6 months |

Fig. 2.1 Main imaging features

Table 2.2 Ancillary imaging features [4]

Favoring malignancy, non HCC in particular	Favoring benignity	Favoring HCC in particular
1- Subthreshold growth (see "threshold growth" in the major criteria section)	1-Size stability ≥2 years	1-Nonenhancing "capsule"
2- Corona enhancement	2-Size reduction	2-Nodule-in-nodule architecture
3- Fat sparing in a solid mass	3-Homogeneous marked T2 hyperintensity	3-Mosaic architecture
4- Restricted diffusion	4-Homogeneous marked T2 or T2* hypointensity	4-Fat in mass, more than adjacent liver
5- Mild-moderate T2 hyperintensity	5-Undistorted vessels	5-Blood products in mass
6- Iron sparing in a solid mass	6-Parallels blood pool enhancement	
7- Transitional phase hypointensity	7-Hepatobiliary phase isointensity	
8- Hepatobiliary phase hypointensity		

Application of CT/MRILI-RADS in Treatment Response Assessment

- **LI-RADS-Treated Categories:**
  - a. *LR-TR-Nonevaluable:* Unable to interpret due to image degradation
  - b. *LR-TR-Nonviable:* No viable tumor tissue suspected
  - c. *LR-TR-Equivocal:* Atypical imaging features for residual tumor tissue

Tables 2.3 and 2.4, respectively. Figure 2.2 depicts a clinical case.

2.2.5 Assigning LI-RADS Categories

- Using the ACR table [3], the main LI-RADS categories can be assigned based on major imaging features.
- LI-RADS categories can be further refined by utilizing ancillary imaging features.

Table 2.3 Evidence-based statistics. What is the percentage of HCC and malignancy associated with each LI-RADS category?

LR-1	LR-2	LR-3	LR-4	LR-5	LR-M
0% HCC, 0% malignancy	16% HCC, 18% malignancy	37% HCC, 39% malignancy	74% HCC, 81% malignancy	95% HCC, 98% malignancy	37% HCC, 94% malignancy

Table 2.4 Common pitfalls [5]

Pitfall	Applying LI-RADS to the wrong patient population	Interpreting hypointensity on transitional-hepatobiliary phase MR images as "washout" appearance	Interpreting any/all peri-observation enhancement as a "capsule"	Not using the LR-M category	Classifying any vascular thrombosis as the tumor in vein
Solution	LI-RADS system should be applied only to a high-risk population	The presence of "washout" should be assessed only on the images acquired during the portal venous phase	Carefully scrutinizing the appearance of peri-observational enhancement on the dynamic study permits a correct interpretation and use of the major feature, "capsule"	A liver observation presenting with a targetoid appearance should be classified as LR-M	TIV should only be applied when the features are unequivocal

- Each benign ancillary feature can down-categorize by one, including from LR-5 to LR-4.
- Each malignant ancillary feature can up-categorize by one, except no up-categorizing from LR-4 to LR-5.

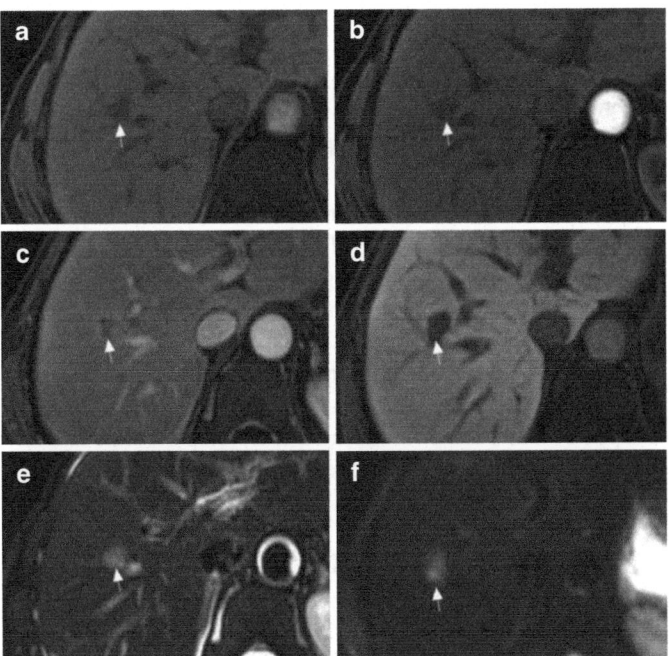

Fig. 2.2 Gadoxetate acid-enhanced magnetic resonance images in a 50-year-old man with hepatitis B-induced liver cirrhosis. (**a**) Pre-contrast magnetic resonance images indicated a 16-mm nodule (arrow) in the right lobe of the liver. (**b**) The nodule was indicated to be hypointense in the hepatic arterial phase; (**c**) to have a washout appearance with the absence of a capsule in the portal venous phase; (**d**) hypointense in the hepatobiliary phase. The nodule was categorized according to Liver Imaging Reporting and Data System 4 with ancillary findings of (**e**) mild-moderate T2 hyper-intensity and (**f**) restricted diffusion [6]

2.2.6 Application of CT/MRI LI-RADS in Treatment Response Assessment

- *LI-RADS-treated categories:*

  (a) *LR-TR-Nonevaluable: Unable to interpret due to image degradation*

  (b) *LR-TR-Nonviable: No viable tumor tissue suspected*

  (c) *LR-TR-Equivocal: Atypical imaging features for residual tumor tissue*

2.3 O-RADS

2.3.1 Definition

2.3.1.1 O-RADS: Ovarian-Adnexal Reporting and Data System

A quality assurance tool for the standardized description of ovarian/adnexal pathology [7]. In the case of the adnexal mass, the correct interpretation leading to the correct diagnosis is the key to accuracy in determining the risk of malignancy and, finally, optimal patient management [7]. Since ultrasound is widely considered the primary imaging modality in evaluating adnexal masses and MRI the problem-solving tool, parallel working groups (US and MRI) were formed to develop separate but consistent groups of terms specific to each modality.

2.3.2 Applicable Population

- O-RADS assumes an average risk patient with no acute symptoms. Clinical management directed by the treating physician would supersede management recommendations based on imaging alone.
- Each patient will be categorized as pre- or postmenopausal, with the postmenopause category defined as amenorrhea of ≥1 year.
- In multiple or bilateral lesions, each lesion should be separately characterized, and management is driven by the lesion with the highest O-RADS score.

O-RADS has six categories, as provided below. Evidence-based statistics is shown in Table 2.5.

Table 2.5 Evidence-based statistics

Positive predictive value (PPV) for malignancy			
O-RADS 2	O-RADS 3	O-RADS 4	O-RADS 5
<0.5%	~5%	~50%	~90%

2.3.3 **Categories** [8]

- **O-RADS 0**: An incomplete evaluation
- **O-RADS 1**: Physiologic category (normal premenopausal ovary)
  - Ovarian follicle or hemorrhagic cyst (<3 cm)
  - Corpus luteum (<3 cm)
- **O-RADS 2**: Almost certainly benign category (<1% risk of malignancy)
  - Simple cyst 3–5 cm
    - Premenopausal: No follow-up
    - Postmenopausal: 1-year follow-up
  - Simple cyst 5–10 cm
    - Premenopausal: 8–12 week follow-up
    - Postmenopausal: 1-year follow-up
  - Nonsimple but unilocular cyst with smooth margins <3 cm
    - Premenopausal: No follow-up
    - Postmenopausal: 1-year follow up if referring to ultrasound specialist or MRI, management by a gynecologist
  - Nonsimple but unilocular cyst with smooth margins 3–10 cm
    - Premenopausal: 8–12 week follow-up
    - Postmenopausal: Refer to ultrasound specialist or MRI; management by a gynecologist
  - Lesions with "classical ultrasound characteristics" of the following but may have specific recommendations:
    - Typical hemorrhagic cyst
    - Dermoid cyst
    - Endometrioma
    - Para-ovarian cyst
    - Peritoneal inclusion cyst
    - Hydrosalpinx
  - Lesion with lipid content and no enhancing solid tissue (MRI)
  - Homogeneously hypointense on T2 and DWI lesion (MRI)

- **O-RADS 3 (Fig. 2.3)**: Low risk of malignancy (1 to <10%)—needs a referral to ultrasound specialist or gynecologist with a view to MRI
  - Unilocular >10 cm (simple or nonsimple)
  - Lesions looking like typical dermoids, endometriomas, or hemorrhagic cysts >10 cm
  - Solid smooth lesion of any with color score 1
  - Multilocular cyst <10 cm smooth inner wall with color score 1–3
  - Lesion with solid tissue (excluding T2 dark/DWI dark); low-risk time-intensity curve on DCE MRI
  - Dilated fallopian tube—nonsimple fluid: thin wall/folds; simple fluid: thick, smooth wall/folds; no enhancing solid tissue (MRI)
- **O-RADS 4**: Lesions with an intermediate risk of malignancy (10 to <50%)—needs ultrasound specialist review or MRI as well as management by a gynecologist with gynecological oncology support or solely by a gynecological oncologist
  - Unilocular cyst with a solid component, any size, 1–3 papillary projections, any color score

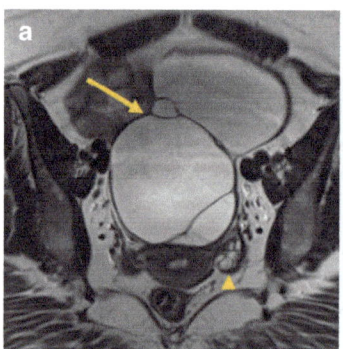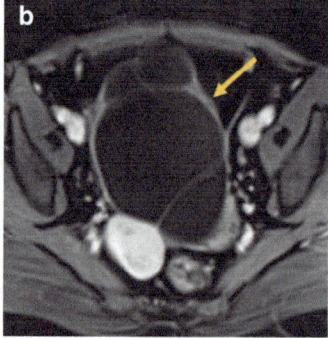

Fig. 2.3 Axial T2WI and delayed postcontrast axial T1WI show a 14.8-cm multilocular right adnexal cyst (arrows) with thin enhancing septations in a 33-year-old premenopausal woman. (**a**) axial T2-weighted image. (**b**) axial T1-weighted image with fat saturation post-contrast. The left ovary is normal (arrowhead). Per O-RADS MRI risk stratification, this is considered an O-RADS 3 (low-risk of malignancy). This patient went on to surgical resection, and pathology confirmed benign serous cystadenofibroma [10]

- Multilocular cyst with a solid component, any size, color score 1–3
- Multilocular cyst without solid component
- >10 cm, smooth inner wall with a color score of 1–3
- Any size smooth inner wall with a color score of 4
- Any size with an irregular inner wall or irregular septations of any color score
- Solid smooth lesion of any with a color score of 2–3
- Lesion with solid tissue (excluding T2 dark/DWI dark); intermediate risk time-intensity curve on DCE MRI; if DCE MRI is not feasible, score 4 is any lesion with solid tissue (excluding T2 dark/DWI dark) that is enhancing ≤myometrium at 30–40 s on non-DCE MR
- Lesion with lipid content; large enhancing solid tissue (MRI)

- **O-RADS 5**: Lesions with a high risk of malignancy (≥50%)—needs a referral to a gynecological oncologist
  - Presence of ascites/peritoneal nodularity
  - Unilocular cyst with papillary projections
  - Multilocular cyst with a solid component
  - Solid lesion—some criteria apply—color score 4
  - Solid irregular lesion of any size
  - Lesion with solid tissue (excluding T2 dark/DWI dark); high-risk time-intensity curve on DCE MRI; if DCE MRI is not feasible, score 5 is any lesion with solid tissue (excluding T2 dark/DWI dark) that is enhancing > myometrium at 30–40 s on non-DCE MRI

2.3.4 Common Pitfalls [9]

- *US Pitfall-1:* The size of the lesion should be obtained by measuring the largest diameter of the lesion regardless of the plane in which that diameter appears.
- *US Pitfall-2:* O-RADS applies only to lesions involving the ovaries and/or fallopian tube. If a pelvic lesion origin is indeterminate but suspected to be ovarian or fallopian in origin, the O-RADS system may apply.

- *US Pitfall-3:* Recommendations are generally based upon transvaginal sonography, although they may be augmented by transabdominal or transrectal sonography as needed.
- *MR Pitfall-1:* Characteristic benign mature teratoma should be scored as O-RADS MRI 2 due to the very low risk of malignancy. Characteristic benign mature teratomas may contain septations or minimal enhancement of Rokitansky nodules, and these findings do not upgrade the lesion to O-RADS MRI Score 4. However, fatty adnexal lesions that contain a large amount of enhancing soft tissue are classified as O-RADS MRI Score 4 due to the risk of immature teratoma or other malignant tissue.
- *MR Pitfall-2:* Some characteristic lesions (e.g., dysgerminoma, granulosa cell tumor, lymphoma, serous papillary tumors, peritoneal pseudocyst) can be confidently diagnosed on MRI regardless of the O-RADS MRI Score category.
- *MR Pitfall-3:* Dynamic contrast enhancement (DCE) with perfusion time-intensity curves are preferred over nondynamic DCE post-contrast imaging for risk assessment. DCE time resolution should be of 15 s or less.

2.4   PI-RADS

2.4.1   Definition

2.4.1.1 PI-RADS (Prostate Imaging–Reporting and Data System)

PI-RADS is a structured reporting scheme for multiparametric prostate MRI (mpMRI) to evaluate suspected prostate cancer in the treatment of native prostate glands [11]. The last version 2.1 was published in 2019 and developed by an internationally representative group involving the American College of Radiology (ACR), the European Society of Urogenital Radiology (ESUR), and AdMeTech.

2.4.2 When Should PI-RADS Be Used?

Multiparametric prostate MRI (mpMRI) of the prostate is primarily used to evaluate prostatic lesions and stratify changes in patients with suspected prostate cancer. PI-RADS assessment uses a 5-point scale based on the probability that a combination of mpMRI findings on T2W, DWI, and DCE correlates with the presence of a clinically significant cancer for each lesion in the prostate gland.

2.4.3 Technical Remarks

PI-RADS can be applied to the following modality:

– Multiparametric magnetic resonance imaging (mpMRI)

PI-RADS has several categories (Table 2.6), with an anatomical sequence-based five-point scale (Table 2.7). Evidence-based statistics and common pitfalls are provided in Tables 2.8 and 2.9, respectively. Figure 2.4 depicts a clinical case.

2.5 Lung-RADS

2.5.1 Definition

2.5.1.1 Lung-RADS: Lung Imaging-Reporting and Data System

Lung-RADS is a classification proposed to aid with findings in low-dose CT (LDCT) lung cancer screening exams and developed by the American College of Radiology (ACR) [15]. The goal of Lung-RADS is to standardize the follow-up and management decisions [16]. The latest version of Lung-RADS is 1.1 and released in 2019.

Table 2.6 PI-RADS categories [12]

PI-RADS 1	PI-RADS 2	PI-RADS 3	PI-RADS 4	PI-RADS 5
Very low (clinically significant cancer is *highly unlikely* to be present)	Low (clinically significant cancer is *unlikely* to be present)	Intermediate (Fig. 2.4) (the presence of clinically significant cancer is *equivocal*)	High (clinically significant cancer is *likely* to be present)	Very high (clinically significant cancer is *highly likely* to be present)

2.5.2 When Should It Be Used?

The Lung-RADS classification is used in describing LDCT in lung cancer screening (for example, NLST), which allows patients to be categorized depending on the presence and size of the lung nodule [17].

Lung-RADS can be applied to the following modalities:

• LDCT for lung cancer screening

2.5.3 Avoid Using Lung-RADS in the Following Populations

• Patients under 55 and over 75 years of age
• Not current or not former smoker with at least a 30 pack-year history of smoking
• Patient with a personal history of lung cancer

Lung-RADS has several categories (Table 2.10), with main imaging features (Table 2.11). Evidence-based statistics and common pitfalls are provided in Tables 2.12 and 2.13, respectively. Figure 2.5 depicts a clinical case.

Table 2.7 Five-point scale for each category and MR sequence

Scale	T2W for TZ	T2W for PZ	DWI	Dynamic contrast enhancement (DCE)
1	• Normal appearing transition zone (rare) or • A round, completely encapsulated nodule ("typical nodule" of benign prostatic hyperplasia)	• Uniform high signal intensity (normal)	• No abnormality on ADC or • High b-value DWI	–
2	• A mostly encapsulated nodule or • A homogeneous circumscribed nodule without encapsulation ("atypical nodule"), or • A homogeneous mildly hypointense area between nodules	• A linear or wedge-shaped hypointensity or • Diffuse mild hypointensity, usually indistinct margin	• A linear/wedge-shaped hypointensity on ADC and/or • A hyperintensity on high b-value DWI	

(continued)

Table 2.7 (continued)

Scale	T2W for TZ	T2W for PZ	DWI	Dynamic contrast enhancement (DCE)
3	• A heterogeneous signal intensity with obscured margins; includes others that do not qualify as 2, 4, or 5	• A heterogeneous signal intensity or • A noncircumscribed, rounded, moderate hypointensity; includes others that do not qualify as 2, 4, or 5	• A focal (discrete and different from background), mild/moderate hypointensity on ADC and/or • A mild/moderate hyperintensity on high b-value DWI; may be markedly hypointense on ADC or markedly hyperintense on high b-value DWI, but not both	• A negative (no early or contemporaneous enhancement, or diffuse multifocal enhancement not corresponding to a focal finding on T2W and/or • DWI, or focal enhancement corresponding to a lesion demonstrating features of benign prostatic hyperplasia on T2W (including features of extruded benign prostatic hyperplasia nodule in the peripheral zone)
4	• A lenticular or noncircumscribed, homogeneous, moderately hypointense, and <1.5 cm in greatest dimension	• A circumscribed, homogeneous, moderate hypointensity, and <1.5 cm in greatest dimension	• A circumscribed, homogeneous, moderate hypointensity, and <1.5 cm in greatest dimension	• A positive (focal, and earlier than or contemporaneous with the enhancement of adjacent normal prostatic tissues, and corresponds to suspicious finding on T2 and/or DWI)

| 5 | • Same as 4, but ≥1.5 cm in greatest dimension or definite extraprostatic extension/invasive behavior | • Same as 4 but ≥1.5 cm in greatest dimension or definite extraprostatic extension/invasive behavior | • Same as 4 but ≥1.5 cm in greatest dimension or definite extraprostatic extension/invasive behavior |

WI weighted imaging; *TZ* transition zone; *PZ* peripheral zone; *DWI* diffusion-weighted imaging; *DCE* dynamic contrast enhancement

Table 2.8 Evidence-based statistics. What is the estimated overall PPV (%) for each category?

PI-RADS 2	PI-RADS 3	PI-RADS 4	PI-RADS 5
>5%	>15%	>39%	>72%

2.6 BI-RADS

2.6.1 Definition

2.6.1.1 BI-RADS: Breast Imaging-Reporting and Data System

BI-RADS aims to provide breast imaging terminology and report structure for mammography, breast ultrasound, and magnetic resonance imaging, resulting in improved communication between clinician and radiologist.

BI-RADS may be used with multiple modalities (Table 2.14) and has several categories (Table 2.15). Reporting considerations are shown in Table 2.16. Evidence-based statistics and common pitfalls are provided in Tables 2.17 and 2.18, respectively. Figure 2.6 depicts a clinical case.

2.7 TI-RADS

2.7.1 Definition

2.7.1.1 TI-RADS: Thyroid Imaging-Reporting and Data System

TI-RADS aims to provide thyroid imaging terminology and report structure for ultrasound, resulting in improved communication between clinicians and radiologists.

2.7.2   Technical Remarks

- Nodules should be measured in three axes: *maximum* dimension on an axial image, *maximum* dimension perpendicular to the previous measurement on the same image, and *maximum* longitudinal dimension on a sagittal image.
- Measurements should also *include* the nodule's *halo* if present.
- No more than *four nodules* with the highest ACR TI-RADS point scores *that fall below the size threshold for FNA* should be followed, as detailed reporting of more than four nodules would needlessly complicate and lengthen reports [25].
- Significant enlargement is defined as a *20% increase* in at least *two* nodule *dimensions* and a minimal increase of *2 mm*, or a *50%* or greater increase in *volume*, as in the criteria adopted by other professional societies [26].

TI-RADS has multiple ultrasonographic features (Fig. 2.7) and utilizes a five-point scale (Table 2.19) with further management recommendations (Table 2.20). Evidence-based statistics is provided in Table 2.21. Figure 2.8 depicts the typical ultrasonographic features of each category.

2.7.3   Common Pitfalls

"Punctate echogenic foci" can encompass both microcalcifications and inspissated colloid, depending on the technique and size of the colloid foci in a nodule. Unlike microcalcifications, foci of an inspissated colloid are not associated with malignancy, and they often appear differently to microcalcifications on closer inspection. An inspissated colloid is not a high-risk feature.

Table 2.9 Common pitfalls [13]

Pitfall	Solution
Hypertrophic anterior fibromuscular stroma	The presence of muscle cells and connective tissue in the most anterior part of the gland, between the two lobes that constitute the TZ
Periprostatic neurovascular bundle	The periprostatic vascular plexus courses around the lateral margins of the prostate and can show a congested appearance, particularly in men with prostatitis
Bilateral benign prostatic hyperplasia proliferation (mustache sign)	The presence of median symmetric, bilateral areas of low signal intensity on T2-WI at the base/middle of the prostate on either side of the ejaculatory ducts can mimic cancer
Median posterior BPH proliferation (teardrop sign)	The presence of a focal/nodular, hypointense area at the middle third or the base (adjacent to the ejaculatory ducts) of the PZ of the prostate could mimic cancer
Prostatitis	Prostatitis is usually caused by *E. coli* or *Staphylococcus* infections and can ultimately result in an abscess
Ectopic BPH nodule	The presence of an ectopic, focal peripheral nodule characterized by low signal intensity on T2-WI, with sharply defined margins, restricted diffusion, and enhancement similar to the central portion of the hypertrophied TZ, could be erroneously interpreted as PCa in the PZ
Abscess vs. cancer	In the PZ, it is possible to find a round-shaped region characterized by inhomogeneous, low-signal intensity on T2-WI, with a pseudo-capsule (scored as 2/5), together with ring enhancement on DCE (+) and restriction on DWI (scored as 4/5)
Hemorrhage	The presence of hemorrhage after a prostate biopsy is relatively frequent. The prostate normally produces citrate for preserving the semen, but it is also an endogenous anticoagulant that can lead to prolonged bleeding and noncoagulation of blood after the biopsy
Focal atrophy	The post-atrophic hyperplastic subtype may mimic PCa on mpMRI due to the glandular crowding and complex architecture

Table 2.9 (continued)

Pitfall	Solution
Necrosis	Necrosis can be seen after the abscess resolution and florid inflammatory changes from infectious prostatitis or after focal therapy
Calcification	Calcification is due to concreted prostatic secretions, calcified corpora amylacea, and phleboliths in the periprostatic venous plexus

2.8   NI-RADS

2.8.1   Definition

2.8.1.1   NI-RADS: Neck Imaging-Reporting and Data System

It is a risk classification for reporting surveillance imaging of the treated head and neck cancer. The terminology and categories may be applied to any head and neck malignancy.

NI-RADS was developed to address whether or not imaging demonstrates evidence of tumor recurrence [28].

NI-RADS is intended for CT, MRI, and PET/CT (Table 2.22) and has five categories (Table 2.23), with CT imaging findings (Table 2.24) as well as PET features (Table 2.25). Evidence-based statistics and management recommendations are provided in Tables 2.26 and 2.27, respectively. Figure 2.9 depicts a clinical case.

2.8.2   Common Pitfalls

- If the primary tumor is near or involving the skull base, MRI should be used instead of CT neck to evaluate soft tissue/perineural involvement.
- When there is discordance between CT and PET, the NI-RADS category should be assigned to the lower adjacent scores.

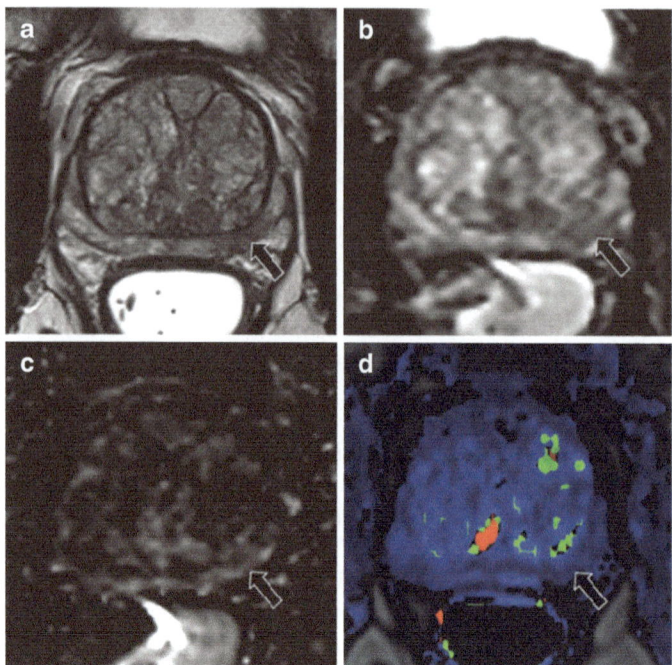

Fig. 2.4 Images of a 67-year-old man with an elevated PSA level (8.7 ng/mL) who had undergone two previous prostate biopsies with normal findings. (**a**) Axial T2-weighted MR image shows a hypointense focal abnormality (arrow) with noncircumscribed margins in the left posterolateral peripheral zone at the midgland, abutting the prostate capsule but without evidence of extraprostatic extension (T2-weighted imaging score: 3). (**b, c**) ADC map (**b**) and computed high-b value (1500 s/mm^2) diffusion-weighted MR image (**c**) show a 1.2-cm lesion that is moderately hypointense on the ADC map (arrow on **b**) and mildly hyperintense on the diffusion-weighted MR image (arrow on **c**) (DWI-ADC score: 3). (**d**) Axial dynamic contrast-enhanced T1-weighted MR image with color-coded overlay (normal enhancement coded in blue) shows no early enhancement (arrow) to correspond with the abnormality seen at T2-weighted MR imaging and DWI-ADC (dynamic contrast-enhanced MR imaging: negative). Because DWI-ADC is the dominant parameter for peripheral zone abnormalities, this focal lesion was assigned a PI-RADS assessment category of 3. The findings at software-based MR imaging/US fusion-guided biopsy of the lesion disclosed prostate cancer with a Gleason score of 3 + 3 [14]

Table 2.10 Lung-RADS categories

Lung-RADS 1	Lung-RADS 2	Lung-RADS 3	Lung-RADS 4a	Lung-RADS 4b/4x
Negative	Benign appearance	Probably benign	Probably suspicious	Suspicious

- Only when CT and PET are concordant for highly suspicious features is the NI-RADS category 3 assigned.

2.9   CAD-RADS

2.9.1   Definition

2.9.1.1 Coronary Artery Disease Imaging-Reporting and Data System

It is a standardized communication method of findings and a clinical decision aid of Coronary CT angiography [31].

CAD-RADS is applicable in two clinical presentations (Table 2.28), with different interpretation categories (Table 2.29) as well as management recommendations (Table 2.30). Evidence-based statistics and common pitfalls are provided in Tables 2.3 and 2.4, respectively. Figure 2.10 depicts a clinical case.

2.9.2   Common Pitfalls

If more than one modifier is present, the symbol "/" (slash) should follow each modifier in the following order:

- Modifier N: nondiagnostic
- Modifier S: stent
- Modifier G: graft
- Modifier V: vulnerability

Table 2.11 Main features for each Lung-RADS category [18]

Category 0	Prior CT studies were performed but are not available for comparison Lungs were incompletely imaged
Category 1 Continue with annual screening	No lung nodules
Category 2 Continue with annual screening	Lung nodule(s) with specific findings favoring benign nodule(s) (complete calcification, central or popcorn calcifications, calcification in concentric rings, fat-containing nodules)
	Solid nodule(s) <6 mm at baseline OR new nodule <4 mm
	Subsolid nodule(s) <6 mm on the baseline screening
	Ground glass nodule(s) <30 mm OR ≥30 mm and unchanged OR slowly growing category 3 or 4 nodules that are unchanged for ≥3 months
Category 3 (Fig. 2.5) 6-month follow-up with LDCT	*Solid* nodule(s) ≥6 mm to <8 mm at baseline OR new nodule 4 mm to <6 mm
	Subsolid nodule(s) ≥6 mm total diameter with solid component <6 mm OR new <6 mm total diameter
	Ground glass nodule(s) ≥30 mm on baseline CT OR new <6 mm total diameter
Category 4A 3-month follow-up with LDCT or PET/CT may be used if there is a ≥8-mm solid component	*Solid* nodule(s) ≥8 mm to <15 mm at baseline OR growing nodule(s) <8 mm OR new nodule 6 mm to <8 mm

Table 2.11 (continued)

Category 0	Prior CT studies were performed but are not available for comparison Lungs were incompletely imaged
	Subsolid nodule(s) with ≥6 mm total diameter of solid component ≥6 mm to <8 mm OR new or growing <4 mm solid component
Category 4B 3-month follow-up with LDCT or PET/CT may be used if there is a ≥8-mm solid component	*Solid* nodule(s) ≥8 mm to <15 mm at baseline OR growing nodule(s) <8 mm OR new nodule 6 mm to <8 mm
	Subsolid nodule(s) with ≥6 mm total diameter of solid component ≥6 mm to <8 mm OR new or growing <4 mm solid component
	Endobronchial nodule
Category 4X Chest CT and/or appropriate PET-CT and/or tissue sampling depending on the probability of malignancy and comorbidities	*Solid* nodule(s) ≥15 mm at baseline new OR growing, and ≥8 mm
	Subsolid nodule(s) with solid component ≥8 mm new OR growing ≥4 mm solid component
	For new large nodules that develop on an annual repeat screening CT, a 1-month LDCT may be recommended to address potentially infectious or inflammatory conditions

Table 2.12 Evidence-based statistics

Categories:	Categories 1 and 2	Category 3	Category 4A	Category 4B/4X
Chance of malignancy:	<1%	1–2%	5–15%	>15%

Table 2.13 Pearls and pitfalls. M. D. Martin et al. identified 15 clinical scenarios with pitfalls of Lung-RADS 1.0, which are actual for Lung-RADS version 1.1 [19]

Common pitfalls	Clinical example
New Lung-RADS category 3 (probably benign) solid lung nodule in an aging patient out of the screening program	An 80-year-old man undergoes the last annual LDCT, which revealed a new 5-mm solid lung nodule (Lung-RADS 3), but in 3 months, the patient will be 81 years old (exclusion criteria from screening)
Lung mass in a patient with vague symptoms	Primary LDCT revealed a 39-mm mass in a 63-year-old patient. A retrospective analysis of the electronic medical record showed that the patient complained of neck pain for the first time
Solid suspicious (Lung-RADS category 4B) nodule with a very slow growth rate	A 74-year-old female patient was diagnosed with a 19-mm solid lung nodule during primary LDCT. CT of the abdominal cavity was performed 12 years ago, and its size was 11 mm. This lung node should be assigned the Lung-RADS 4B category based on the size and growth dynamics
Ground-glass nodule that increases in density but remains stable in size	A 66-year-old patient was found to have a ground glass nodule, and a follow-up study showed an increase in its density without pronounced size dynamics. What Lung-RADS category should be assigned in this situation?
Ground-glass nodule with a slow growth rate	Lung-RADS 2 category includes lung nodules and ground glass nodules less than 30 mm or 30 mm or more with size stability/very slow growth rate. The exact definition of the latter term is not available in the current version of Lung-RADS
How to measure and classify a part-solid nodule	The division into solid and subsolid pulmonary nodules is subjective and varies greatly
Nodule that decreases in size but increases in attenuation	Lung-RADS is not currently considering decreasing the size of the pulmonary nodules

Table 2.13 (continued)

Common pitfalls	Clinical example
Incidental potentially important finding other than lung cancer detected at low-dose LCS CT	Incidental findings detected in diagnostic imaging studies are common and are among the criticisms of low-dose CT for LCS. However, the ACR does not define a "clinically" or "potentially" significant finding, leaving the interpretation of the term to the radiologist
Categorization of a cavitary lung nodule or nodules	Many conditions can manifest as solitary or multiple cavitary nodules, including lung cancer, metastasis, infection, granulomatosis with polyangiitis, and pulmonary Langerhans cell histiocytosis. Lung-RADS does not address the categorization and management of cavitary lung nodules
Low-dose LCS CT of a patient with a treated low-risk nonlung malignancy	Should a 62-year-old woman treated for stage I breast cancer 18 months ago who is eligible for LCS undergo LCS CT? Current recommendations do not address patients who have been treated for nonlung malignancies, including those with a low risk of recurrence

2.10   C-RADS

2.10.1 Definition

2.10.1.1   CT Colonography Reporting and Data System

C-RADS aims to standardize the reporting of colorectal and extra-colonic findings in CT colonography (CTC) [33]. Assessment categories reflect lesion morphology, size, and number. Beyond improved communication between radiologists and physicians, the classification complements clinical research, quality assessment, and patient outcomes. C-RADS includes different categories for colonic and extra-colonic findings. Due to its ability to simultaneously screen for colorectal cancer and abdominal aortic aneurysm, CTC is a highly cost-effective and clinically efficacious screening strategy [34].

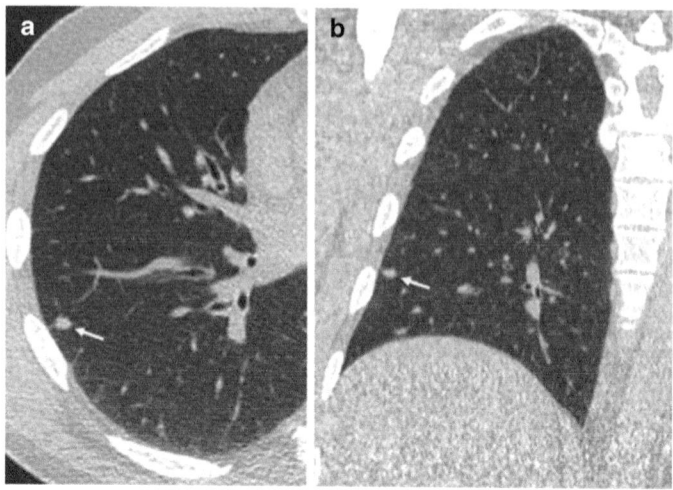

Fig. 2.5 Images show lung cancer screening CT scan in a 57-year-old man. (**a**) Axial and (**b**) coronal images show right lower-lobe nodule (arrow) classified as Lung CT Screening Reporting and Data System (Lung-RADS) category 3 nodule by all readers using manual measurements and as Lung-RADS 2 nodule by all readers using volumetry. The manual average diameter is 7 mm as measured by two readers and 6 mm as measured by one reader; semiautomated average diameter is 6 mm as measured by two readers and 7 mm as measured by one reader; and semiautomated volume is 91 mm³, 96 mm³, and 99 mm³ as measured by each of three readers. Note the relatively flat nonspherical shape in b. Nodule remains stable on subsequent scans up to 2.5 years later [20]

2.10.2 Technical Remarks

Use multidetector CT (MDCT) with pitch/table feed per rotation adjusted to achieve full anatomical coverage within a single breath-hold, minimizing movement artifact [35]. For bowel preparation, full laxation without fecal tagging is the required minimum. Colonic distension with carbon dioxide, preferably using an automated insufflator. Hyoscine butylbromide improving colonic distension is to be actively considered unless contraindicated. An initial "scout" view is used to assess bowel preparation and distension. Radiation dose as low as reasonably

Table 2.14 Technical remarks

US	Mammography	MRI
• Routinely includes B-mode ultrasonography and color Doppler.	• Includes bilateral craniocaudal (CC) and mediolateral oblique (MLO) views [1].	• Provides numerous acceptable methods of image acquisition with guidelines considered to be a reasonable minimum for achieving acceptable image quality.
• Harmonic imaging and compound imaging can be used to optimize the image contrast and resolution [1].	• In patients with recent surgery, limited imaging may be appropriate.	• A dedicated bilateral breast surface coil should be used. Most published studies have been conducted on 1.5T scanners, but there are some reports from 1.0T units [1].
• Elastography is a valuable supplementary tool, as higher mean stiffness values at shear-wave elastography tend to exhibit inferior prognostic features [2]	• Enlarged or painful lesions, the technician could tailor the views after consultation with the radiologist	• The American College of Radiology noted that no single method of image acquisition had been proven superior to others and field strength, pre-contrast and post-contrast sequences used, method of fat suppression, and postprocessing performed should be reported [3].
		• The abbreviated protocol provides functional information on tumor vascularity and may be more suitable for the diagnosis of biologically aggressive cancers while avoiding the diagnosis of indolent disease [2].

Table 2.15 Categories. BI-RADS has seven categories, ranging from incomplete study to biopsy-proven malignancy

BI-RADS 0
• Indicates the need for **additional evaluation** or **prior studies** for comparison.

BI-RADS 1
• **Negative**, symmetrical, and no masses, architectural distortion, or suspicious calcifications.

BI-RADS 2
• **Definitely benign** lesions, including fibroadenoma, lipoma, intramammary lymph node, and simple cyst. Any BI-RADS 2 breast finding is not expected to change over the follow-up interval.

BI-RADS 3
• **Intermediate** findings with malignancy risk up to two percent, reserved for the diagnostic setting, such as when patients are recalled from screening or present with a palpable lump. BI-RADS 3 carries a management recommendation for **short-term follow-up**. Short-term follow-up is to be recommended with modality or modalities that have best demonstrated the initial finding and a typical schedule of **6, 12, and 24 months**. With stability documented for at least two years, the finding can be downgraded to BI-RADS 2 (benign). If the finding develops suspicious features, then it should be upgraded to BI-RADS 4 or 5.

BI-RADS 4
• Suspicious abnormality with a definite **probability** of being **malignant**. This category can be further divided into **4A (low 2-9%)**, **4B (intermediate 10-49%)**, and **4C (moderate 50-94%)**. A biopsy is recommended for these lesions.

BI-RADS 5
• **High-risk (>95%)** lesions, suspicious for **malignancy**. Biopsy and further management are mandatory for this category. The implication of a BI-RADS 5 finding, in contrast to BIRADS 4, is that if the histology is benign, it should be considered discordant with imaging findings, and lesion excision is still advised.

BI-RADS 6
• **Biopsy-proven** malignancy.

practicable: 120 kVp, craniocaudal direction, collimation ≤3 mm, slice thickness ≥1 mm. Dual-position scanning is necessary for CTC; in cases of immobility or obesity, lateral decubitus imaging is an alternative. Review CTC data before the end of the examination to decide if additional scans are required.

C-RADS has several categories for colonic (Table 2.31) and extra-colonic (Table 2.32) findings, with crucial imaging features (Table 2.33). Figure 2.11 depicts a clinical case.

2.10.3 Reporting Algorithm

Study interpretation requires software providing an axial 2D display, multiplanar reformats, and a 3D endoluminal reconstruction. Structured reporting is preferable, possibly in the table form. Consider double reading CTC. CAD may augment reader sensitivity.

Table 2.16 Reporting algorithm. For each modality, the report should include breast tissue composition and presence of masses, including their shape, margin, structure, associated features, and location [21]

US	Mammography	MRI
• Report focuses acoustic pattern, lesion orientation & elasticity with several special cases -simple cyst, clustered microcysts, complicated cyst, skin mass, foreign body, lymph nodes (intramammary or axillary), vascular abnormalities, postsurgical seroma, and fat necrosis.	• Reporting requires lesion density and margin, as well as a detailed outlook on calcifications and architectural distortion.	• Report provides data on background parenchymal enhancement, lesion internal enhancement (including kinetic curve) and margin, non-mass enhancement, or findings. This modality also provides detailed insight into the implants.

Table 2.17 Evidence-based statistics. What is the percentage of malignancy associated with each BI-RADS category? [22]

BI-RADS 2	BI-RADS 3	BI-RADS 4	BI-RADS 5
0%	2%	30%	97%

Table 2.18 Common pitfalls [23]

BI-RADS 0	• Don't use if prior mammography or US are not available, however NOT required to make a final assessment. • Don't use if prior mammography or US are irrelevant, because the finding is already suspicious. • Don't use for findings that warrant further evaluation with MRI, but make a report before the MRI is performed.
BI-RADS 2	• Don't use when a benign finding is present but not described in the report, then use Category 1. • Don't recommend MRI to further evaluate a benign finding.
BI-RADS 3	• Don't use if unsure whether to render a benign (Category 2) or suspicious (Category 4) assessment. Then use Category 4. • Don't use in a screening examination. • Don't use if a lesion, previously assessed as Category 3 has increased in size or extent, like a mass on US with an increase of 20% or more of longest dimension. Then use category 4.
BI-RADS 5	• Don't use if only one highly suspicious finding is present. Then use Category 4c.
BI-RADS 6	• Don't use after attempted surgical excision with positive margins and no imaging findings other than postsurgical scarring. Then use category 2 and add sentence stating the absence of mammographic correlate for the pathology. • Don't use for imaging findings, demonstrating suspicious findings other than the known cancer, then use Category 4 or 5.

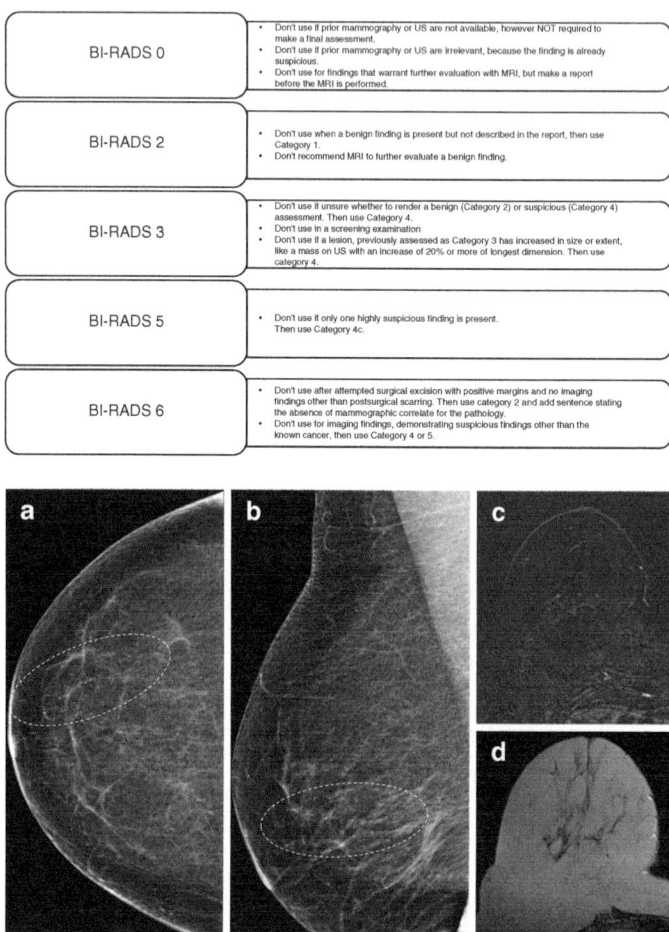

Fig. 2.6 Screening detected segmental linear and coarse heterogeneous microcalcifications BI-RADS 4a in the right breast of a 59-year-old woman (**a**, **b**). Contrast-enhanced MRI (**c**) revealed no enhancing lesions, and small foci were not associated with the microcalcifications. T2-weighted images did not reveal any architectural distortions (**d**). Histopathology revealed secretory changes, B2 [24]

Composition:

- Cystic or completely cystic *:   0 points
- Spongiform *:   0 points
- Mixed cystic and solid: 1 point
- Solid or almost completely solid: 2 points

Echogenicity:

- Anechoic: 0 points
- Hyper-or Isoechoic: 1 point
- Hypoechoic: 2 points
- Very hypoechoic: 3 points

Shape:

- Wider than tall: 0 points
- Taller than wide: 3 points

Margin:

- Smooth: 0 points
- Ill-defined: 0 points
- Lobulated/irregular: 2 points
- Extra-thyroidal extension: 3 points

Echogenic foci:

- None: 0 points
- Large comet-tail artifact: 0 points
- Macrocalcifications: 1 point
- Peripheral/Rim calcifications: 2 points
- Punctate echogenic foci: 3 points

Fig. 2.7 Categories by ultrasonographic features (Fig. 2.8). * Predominantly cystic or spongiform nodules are inherently benign. If these features are present, no further points will be added (automatically TR1)

Table 2.19 Scoring and classification

TR1	TR2	TR3	TR4	TR5
0–1 points	2 points	3 points	4–6 points	≥7 points
Benign	Not suspicious	Mildly suspicious	Moderately suspicious	Highly suspicious

Table 2.20 Recommendations

TR1	TR2	TR3	TR4	TR5
No FNA required	No FNA required	≥15–24 mm follow-up ≥25 mm FNA	≥10–14 mm follow-up ≥15 mm FNA	≥5–9 mm follow-up ≥10 mm FNA
		Follow up: 1, 3, and 5 years	Follow up: 1, 2, 3, and 5 years	Annual follow-up for up to 5 years

Table 2.21 Evidence-based statistics

Categories	TI-RADS 1	TI-RADS 2	TI-RADS 3	TI-RADS 4	TI-RADS 5
Risk of malignancy	0.3%	1.5%	4.8%	9.1%	35%

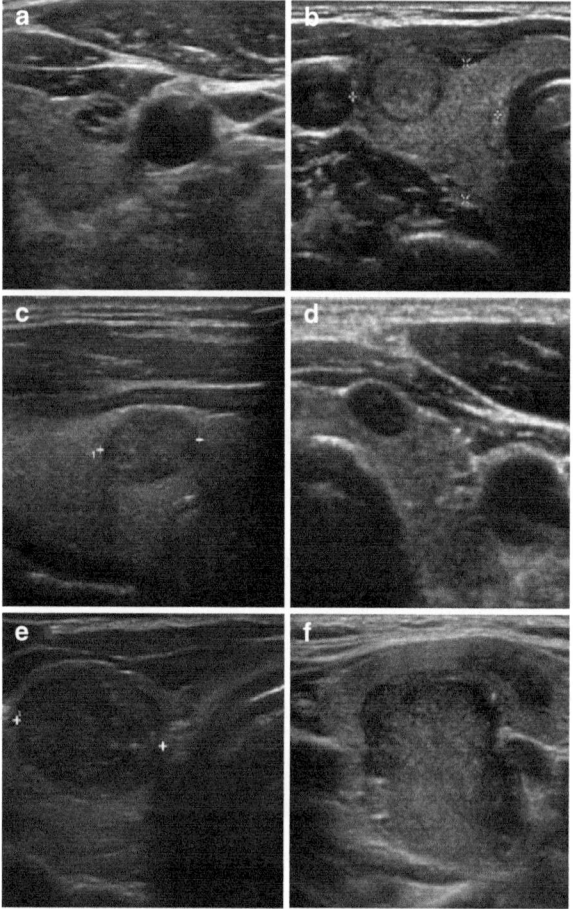

Fig. 2.8 Examples of thyroid nodules submitted to cytological examination. (**a**) Nodule classified as TI-RADS 2; (**b**) TI-RADS 3; (**c**) TI-RADS 4A; (**d**) TI-RADS 4B; (**e**) TI-RADS 4C; (**f**) TI-RADS 5; cases **a**, **b**, and **c** were considered benign; cases **d**, **e**, and **f** were considered malignant according to the Bethesda system [27]

Table 2.22 Technical remarks. NI-RADS is intended for CT, MRI, and 18F-FDG PET/CT. Surveillance may begin as early as 8–12 weeks post-treatment [29]

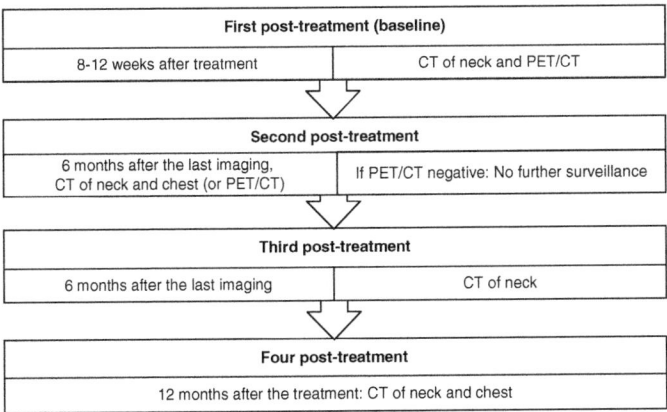

First post-treatment (baseline)	
8-12 weeks after treatment	CT of neck and PET/CT

Second post-treatment	
6 months after the last imaging, CT of neck and chest (or PET/CT)	If PET/CT negative: No further surveillance

Third post-treatment	
6 months after the last imaging	CT of neck

Four post-treatment	
12 months after the treatment: CT of neck and chest	

Table 2.23 Categories

NI-RADS 0	NI-RADS 1	NI-RADS 2	NI-RADS 3	NI-RADS 4
Incomplete (prior imaging unavailable, but will be obtained)	No evidence of recurrence	Low suspicion of recurrence 2a—superficial mucosal (Fig. 2.9) 2b—deep	High suspicion of recurrence ("can and should be biopsied")	Known recurrence

Table 2.24 CT imaging findings

NI-RADS 1	NI-RADS 2	NI-RADS 3

• **Primary site**
  • Expected post-treatment changes with non-mass-like distortion of soft tissues
  • Low-density submucosal/mucosal edema (post-radiation edema)
  • Diffuse curvilinear mucosal enhancement (especially after radiation, i.e. radiation mucositis)
• **Neck**
  • No nodal enlargement or new suspicious morphology (necrosis, extra-nodal extension)
	• **Primary site**
	  • 2a: Non-mass-like, focal, mucosal enhancement
	  • 2b: Non-mass-like, ill-defined, deep soft tissue with only mild differential enhancement
	• **Neck**
	  • Enlarging node(s), without new suspicious morphology (necrosis, extra-nodal extension)
		• **Primary site**
		  • New or enlarging discrete soft tissue with intense differential enhancement
		  • +/- osseous erosion
		• **Neck**
		  • Enlarging node(s), with new necrosis or gross extranodal extension

Table 2.25 PET (FDG) imaging findings

NI-RADS 1	NI-RADS 2	NI-RADS 3

• Primary site
  • No abnormal FDG uptake
  • Diffuse curvilinear mucosal FDG uptake after radiation (benign radiation mucositis)
• Neck
  • No FDG avidity of residual nodes
	• Primary site
	  • 2a: Mild focal mucosal FDG uptake
	  • 2b: Mild FDG uptake to ill-defined deep soft tissue
	• Neck
	  • Mild FDG uptake to residual nodes
		• Primary site
		  • Intense focal FDG uptake to discrete nodule/mass
		• Neck
		  • Intense FDG uptake to residual, new, or enlarging nodes

Table 2.26 Evidence-based statistics [30]

Categories	NI-RADS 1	NI-RADS 2	NI-RADS 3
Risk of malignancy:	4%	15–17%	59%

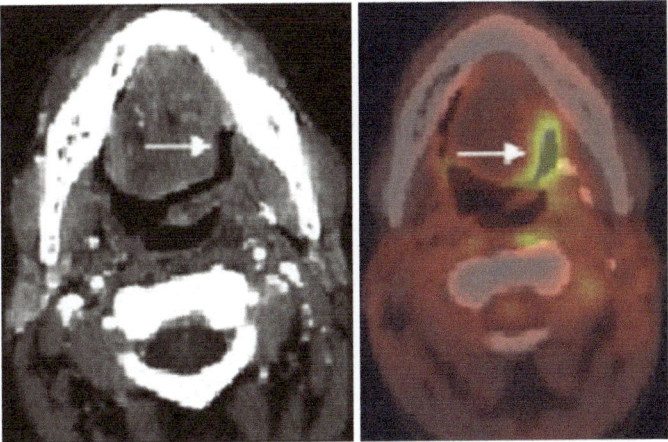

Fig. 2.9 NI-RADS primary 2a: oropharyngeal SCCA treated with CRT. Twelve weeks post-CRT, baseline surveillance PET/CECT shows ulceration along left glossotonsillar sulcus (arrow) without deep enhancement or other concerning features on CECT. However, PET shows intense focal uptake in this region (arrow). Although anatomic appearance on CECT is reassuring, the study is assigned a NI-RADS category 2a so that surgeons look specifically at this area. On direct inspection, this seemed consistent with radiation injury, and follow-up PET was negative [28]

2.10.4 Common Pitfalls

Pitfalls in CTC reporting can be related to technique and anatomy [36]. The former includes retained solid fecal material or luminal fluid, inadequate colon distention or imaging artifacts, polyp contrast coating, 2D-only detection, and measurement pitfalls. The latter pitfall group includes thickened folds, diverticula, flat/submucosal/extrinsic lesions, and anorectal/ileocecal/appendiceal location.

Table 2.27 Management recommendations

NI-RADS 0	NI-RADS 1	NI-RADS 2a	NI-RADS 2b	NI-RADS 3	NI-RADS 4
• Obtain prior imaging examinations, after which a score can be assigned in an addendum	• Continue routine surveillance	• Direct visual inspection of the area of concern	• Additional PET or • Short-interval (3 months) follow-up with CT	• Biopsy (image-guided or clinical) area of concern	• Treatment of disease (with or without biopsy)

Table 2.28 Applicable population. This classification is intended for patients with two different clinical presentations

1- Stable chest pain	2- Acute chest pain, negative first troponin, negative or nondiagnostic electrocardiogram, and low to intermediate risk (Thrombolysis in Myocardial Infarction (TIMI) risk score <4)

Table 2.29 Interpretation categories

1- Stable chest pain	2- Acute chest pain

• **CAD-RADS 0**: Documented **absence** of coronary artery disease
  • **0%** maximal coronary stenosis and no plaques
	• **CAD-RADS 0**: Acute coronary syndrome **highly unlikely**
	  • **0%** maximal coronary stenosis

• **CAD-RADS 1**: **Minimal** nonobstructive coronary artery disease
  • **1-24%** maximal coronary stenosis = minimal stenosis, or plaque with no stenosis (positive remodeling)
	• **CAD-RADS 1**: Acute coronary syndrome **highly unlikely**
	  • **1-24%** maximal coronary stenosis, or plaque with no stenosis (positive remodeling)

• **CAD-RADS 2**: **Mild** nonobstructive coronary artery disease
  • **25-49%** maximal coronary stenosis = mild stenosis
	• **CAD-RADS 2**: **acute coronary syndrome unlikely**
	  • **25-49%** maximal coronary stenosis

• **CAD-RADS 3**: **Moderate** stenosis (**figure 10**)
  • **50-69%** maximal coronary stenosis
	• **CAD-RADS 3**: **acute coronary syndrome possible**
	  • **50-69%** maximal coronary stenosis

• **CAD-RADS 4**: **Severe** stenosis
  • **CAD-RADS 4A**: 70-99% maximal coronary stenosis
  • **CAD-RADS 4B**:**Left main >50%** stenosis or **three-vessel**obstructive (≥70% stenosis) disease
	• **CAD-RADS 4**: **acute coronary syndrome likely**
	  • **CAD-RADS 4A**: 70-99% maximal coronary stenosis
	  • **CAD-RADS 4B**: **Left main >50%** stenosis or **three-vessel**obstructive (≥70% stenosis) disease

• **CAD-RADS 5**: **Total** coronary occlusion
  • **100%** coronary stenosis = total occlusion
	• **CAD-RADS 5**: Acute coronary syndrome **very likely**
	  • **100%** maximal coronary stenosis = total occlusion

• **CAD-RADS N**: Obstructive coronary artery disease **cannot be excluded**
  • Nondiagnostic study
	• **CAD-RADS N**: Acute coronary syndrome **cannot be excluded**
	  • Nondiagnostic study

Table 2.30 Management recommendations

1- Stable chest pain	2- Acute chest pain
CAD-RADS 0 • No further cardiac investigation • Reassurance; consider nonatherosclerotic causes of chest pain	**CAD-RADS 0** • No further evaluation of acute coronary syndrome is required; consider other etiologies
CAD-RADS 1 • No further cardiac investigation • Consider nonatherosclerotic causes of chest pain; consider preventive therapy and risk factor modification	**CAD-RADS 1** • Consider evaluation of non-acute coronary syndrome etiology, if normal troponin and no ECG changes • Consider referral for outpatient follow-up for preventive therapy and risk factor modification
CAD-RADS 2 • No further cardiac investigation • Consider non-atherosclerotic causes of chest pain; consider preventive therapy and risk factor modification, particularly for patients with nonobstructive plaque in multiple segments	**CAD-RADS 2** • Consider evaluation of non-acute coronary syndrome etiology, if normal troponin and no ECG changes • Consider referral for outpatient follow-up for preventive therapy and risk factor modification • If clinical suspicion of acute coronary syndrome is high or if high-risk plaque features are noted, consider hospital admission with cardiology consultation
CAD-RADS 3 • Consider functional assessment • Consider symptom-guided anti-ischemic and preventive pharmacotherapy as well as risk factor modification per guideline-directed care; other treatments should be considered per guideline-directed care	**CAD-RADS 3** • Consider hospital admission with cardiology consultation, functional testing, and/or invasive coronary angiography for evaluation and management. • Recommendation for anti-ischemic and preventive management should be considered as well as risk factor modification; other treatments should be considered if presence of hemodynamically significant lesion.
CAD-RADS 4 • **CAD-RADS 4A:** Consider invasive coronary angiography or functional assessment • **CAD-RADS 4B:** Invasive coronary angiography is recommended • Consider symptom-guided anti-ischemic and preventive pharmacotherapy as well as risk factor modification per guideline-directed care; other treatments (including options of revascularization) should be considered per guideline-directed care	**CAD-RADS 4** • Consider hospital admission with cardiology consultation; further evaluation with invasive coronary angiography and revascularization as appropriate • Recommendation for anti-ischemic and preventive management should be considered as well as risk factor modification
CAD-RADS 5 • Consider invasive coronary angiography and/or viability assessment • Consider symptom-guided anti-ischemic and preventive pharmacotherapy as well as risk factors modification per guideline-directed care;other treatments (including options of revascularization) should be considered per guideline-directed care.	**CAD-RADS 5** • Consider expedited invasive coronary angiography on a timely basis and revascularization if appropriate if acute occlusion • Recommendation for anti-ischemic and preventive management should be considered as well as risk factor modifications.
CAD-RADS N • Additional or alternative evaluation may be needed	**CAD-RADS N** • Additional or alternative evaluation for acute coronary syndrome is needed

Common Pitfalls:

If more than one modifier is present, the symbol "/"(slash) should follow each modifier in the following order:

- Modifier N: nondiagnostic
- Modifier S: stent
- Modifier G: graft
- Modifier V: vulnerability

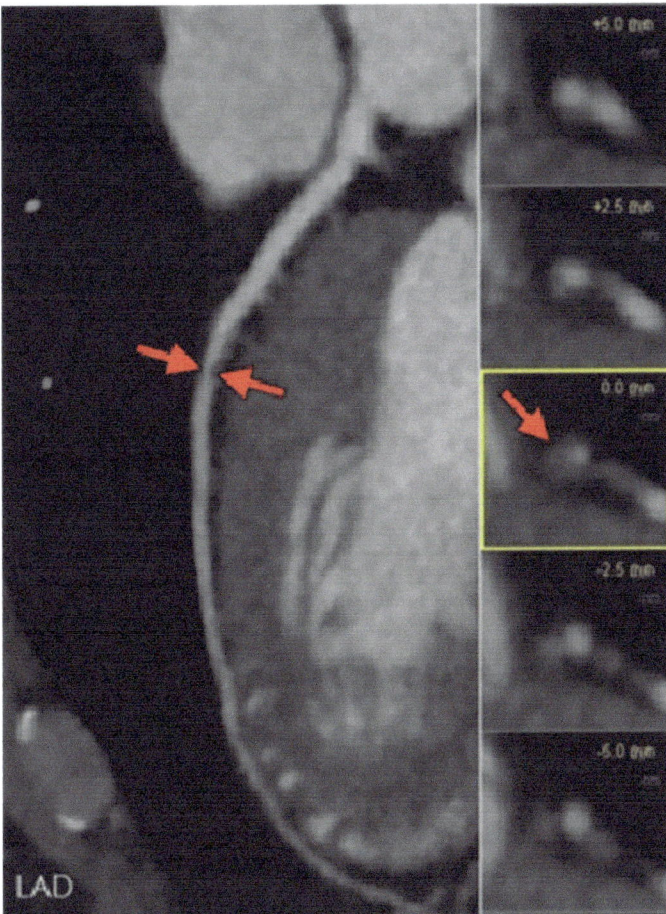

Fig. 2.10 CAD-RADS 3 in a 65-year-old man with atypical chest pain. Curved MPR CT angiographic image (left) and corresponding axial CT images (right) show a noncalcified plaque (arrows) at the mid-LAD artery that is causing moderate stenosis (50%–69%). Functional assessment was recommended. Myocardial perfusion scintigraphy (not shown) showed a stress perfusion defect in the apical anterior and inferior segments, consistent with ischemia [32]

Table 2.31 Categories (colonic findings)

C0 (**Inadequate** study or **previous data** required)
- Lesions ≥10 mm may be obscured due to fluid/feces
- Collapsed colonic segment on both scans
- Previous studies needed for comparison

C1 (**Unremarkable** colon or **benign** finding, follow-up in 5-10 years)
- No visible colonic lesions or abnormalinites
- No polyp ≥6 mm
- Non-neoplastic lesions (e.g. lipoma or diverticulum)

C2 (**Intermediate** risk, proceed with surveillance or colonoscopy)
- Less than 3 polyps from 6 to 9 mm in size
- Unable to exclude a polyp ≥6 mm in an adequate scan

C3 (**Possibly advanced adenoma**, refer to colonoscopy per accepted guidelines for communication)
- Polyp ≥10 mm
- More than 3 polyps from 6 to 9 mm in size

C4 (**Colonic mass**, refer for surgical consultation)
- Bowel lumen compromised
- Extracolonic invasion noted

Table 2.32 Categories (extracolonic findings)

E0 (Evaluation **limited**)

E1 (**Unremarkable** exam or **variant** anatomy)

E2 (**Unimportant** finding, no follow-up required)
- Liver or kidney cysts
- Gallbladder stones
- Vertebral hemangioma

E3 (**Incomplete** characterization, work-up may be required)
- Hyperdense renal cyst

E4 (**Important** finding, communicate to physician)
- Solid renal mass
- Aortic aneurysm
- Solid pulmonary nodule ≥1 cm

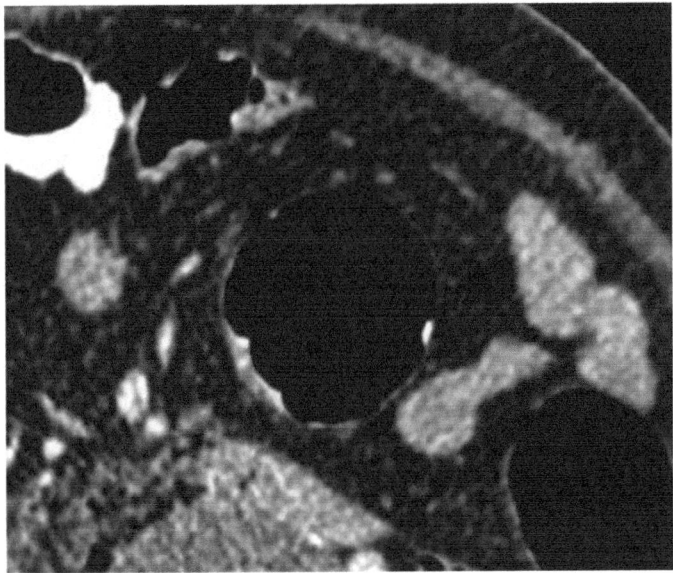

Fig. 2.11 Flat polypoid lesion. According to the C-RADS classification, flat lesions are those lesions that measure 3 mm or less in height [37]

Table 2.33 Findings

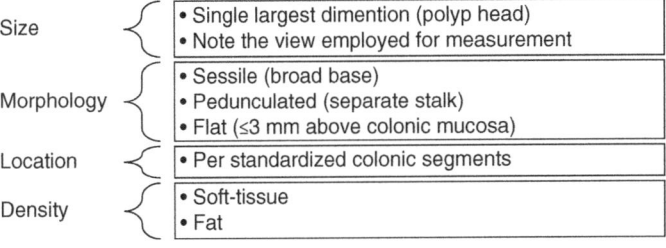

Size	• Single largest dimention (polyp head) • Note the view employed for measurement
Morphology	• Sessile (broad base) • Pedunculated (separate stalk) • Flat (≤3 mm above colonic mucosa)
Location	• Per standardized colonic segments
Density	• Soft-tissue • Fat

References

1. Siedlikowski ST, Kielar AZ, Ormsby EL, Bijan B, Kagay C. Implementation of LI-RADS into a radiological practice. Abdom Radiol. 2018;43(1):179–84.
2. Elsayes KM, et al. White paper of the Society of Abdom Radiol hepatocellular carcinoma diagnosis disease-focused panel on LI-RADS v2018 for CT and MRI. Abdom. Radiol. 2018;43(10):2625–42.
3. van der Pol CB, et al. Accuracy of the liver imaging reporting and data system in computed tomography and magnetic resonance image analysis of hepatocellular carcinoma or overall malignancy—a systematic review. Gastroenterology. 2019;156(4):976–86.
4. Chernyak V, et al. LI-RADS ® ancillary features on CT and MRI. Abdom Radiol. 2018;43(1):82–100.
5. Cannella R, Fowler KJ, Borhani AA, Minervini MI, Heller M, Furlan A. Common pitfalls when using the Liver Imaging Reporting and Data System (LI-RADS): lessons learned from a multi-year experience. Abdom Radiol. 2019;44(1):43–53.
6. Tang Q, Ma C. Performance of gd-eob-dtpa-enhanced mri for the diagnosis of li-rads 4 category hepatocellular carcinoma nodules with different diameters. Oncol Lett. 2018;16(2):2725–31.
7. Ovarian-Adnexal Reporting & Data System | American College of Radiology. [Online]. https://www.acr.org/Clinical-Resources/Reporting-and-Data-Systems/O-Rads. Accessed 21 Dec 2020.
8. Andreotti RF, et al. O-RADS US risk stratification and management system: a consensus guideline from the ACR Ovarian-Adnexal Reporting and Data System Committee. Radiology. 2020;294(1):168–85.
9. Thomassin-Naggara I, et al. Ovarian-Adnexal Reporting Data System Magnetic Resonance Imaging (O-RADS MRI) score for risk stratification of sonographically indeterminate adnexal masses. JAMA Netw Open. 2020;3(1):e1919896.
10. Stein EB, Roseland ME, Shampain KL, Wasnik AP, Maturen KE. Contemporary guidelines for adnexal mass imaging: a 2020 update. Abdom Radiol. 2021;46(5):2127–39.
11. PI-RADS | American College of Radiology. [Online]. https://www.acr.org/Clinical-Resources/Reporting-and-Data-Systems/PI-RADS. Accessed 21 Dec 2020.
12. Westphalen AC, et al. Variability of the positive predictive value of PI-RADS for prostate MRI across 26 centers: experience of the society of Abdom Radiol prostate cancer disease-focused panel. Radiology. 2020;296(1):76–84.
13. Panebianco V, et al. An update of pitfalls in prostate mpMRI: a practical approach through the lens of PI-RADS v. 2 guidelines. Insights Imaging. 2018;9(1):87–101.

14. Purysko AS, Rosenkrantz AB, Barentsz JO, Weinreb JC, Macura KJ. PI-RADS version 2: a pictorial update. Radiographics. 2016;36(5):1354–72.
15. Lung Rads | American College of Radiology. [Online]. https://www.acr.org/Clinical-Resources/Reporting-and-Data-Systems/Lung-Rads. Accessed 21 Dec 2020.
16. Mckee BJ, Regis SM, McKee AB, Flacke S, Wald C. Performance of ACR lung-RADS in a clinical CT lung screening program. J Am Coll Radiol. 2015;12(3):273–6.
17. Callister MEJ, et al. British thoracic society guidelines for the investigation and management of pulmonary nodules. Thorax. 2015;70:ii1–ii54.
18. Fintelmann FJ, et al. The 10 pillars of lung cancer screening: rationale and logistics of a lung cancer screening program. Radiographics. 2015;35(7):1893–908.
19. Martin MD, Kanne JP, Broderick LS, Kazerooni EA, Meyer CA. Lung-RADS: pushing the limits. Radiographics. 2017;37(7):1975–93.
20. Gierada DS, Rydzak CE, Zei M, Rhea L. Improved interobserver agreement on lung-RADS classification of solid nodules using semiautomated CT volumetry. Radiology. 2020;297(3):675–84.
21. Breast Imaging Reporting & Data System | American College of Radiology. [Online]. https://www.acr.org/Clinical-Resources/Reporting-and-Data-Systems/Bi-Rads. Accessed 21 Nov 2020.
22. Orel SG, Kay N, Reynolds C, Sullivan DC. BI-RADS categorization as a predictor of malignancy. Radiology. 1999;211(3):845–50.
23. The Radiology Assistant: Bi-RADS for Mammography and Ultrasound 2013. [Online]. https://radiologyassistant.nl/breast/bi-rads/bi-rads-for-mammography-and-ultrasound-2013. Accessed 21 Nov 2020.
24. Bennani-Baiti B, Dietzel M, Baltzer PA. MRI for the assessment of malignancy in BI-RADS 4 mammographic microcalcifications. PLoS One. 2017;12(11):e0188679.
25. Burch HB, Burman KD, Cooper DS, Hennessey JV, Vietor NO. A 2015 survey of clinical practice patterns in the management of thyroid nodules. J Clin Endocrinol Mctab. 2016;101(7):2853–62.
26. Tessler FN, et al. ACR Thyroid Imaging, Reporting and Data System (TI-RADS): white paper of the ACR TI-RADS Committee. J Am Coll Radiol. 2017;14(5):587–95.
27. Rahal A, et al. Correlation of Thyroid Imaging Reporting and Data System [TI-RADS] and fine needle aspiration: experience in 1,000 nodules. Einstein (Sao Paulo). 2016;14(2):119–23.
28. Aiken AH, et al. ACR Neck Imaging Reporting and Data Systems (NI-RADS): a white paper of the ACR NI-RADS Committee. J Am Coll Radiol. 2018;15(8):1097–108.
29. Aiken AH, et al. Implementation of a novel surveillance template for head and neck cancer: Neck Imaging Reporting and Data System (NI-RADS). J Am Coll Radiol. 2016;13(6):743–746.e1.

30. Wangaryattawanich P, Branstetter BF, Hughes M, Clump DA, Heron DE, Rath TJ. Negative predictive value of NI-RADS category 2 in the first post-treatment FDG-PET/CT in head and neck squamous cell carcinoma. Am J Neuroradiol. 2018;39(10):1884–8.

31. Cury RC, et al. CAD-RADSTM coronary artery disease—reporting and data system. An expert consensus document of the Society of Cardiovascular Computed Tomography (SCCT), the American College of Radiology (ACR) and the North American Society for Cardiovascular Imaging (NASCI). Endorsed by the American College of Cardiology. J Cardiovasc Comput Tomogr. 2016;10(4):269–81.

32. Canan A, Ranganath P, Goerne H, Abbara S, Landeras L, Rajiah P. CAD-RADS: pushing the limits. Radiographics. 2020;40(3):629–52.

33. Zalis ME, et al. CT colonography reporting and data system: a consensus proposal. Radiology. 2005;236(1):3–9.

34. Pickhardt PJ, Hassan C, Laghi A, Kim DH. CT colonography to screen for colorectal cancer and aortic aneurysm in the medicare population: cost-effectiveness analysis. Am J Roentgenol. 2009;192(5):1332–40.

35. Schonberger M, Lefere P, Dachman AH. Pearls and pitfalls of interpretation in CT colonography. Can Assoc Radiol J. 2020;71(2):140–8.

36. Pickhardt PJ, Kim DH. CT colonography. Pitfalls in interpretation. Radiol Clin N Am. 2013;51(1):69–88.

37. Pagés Llinás M, Darnell Martín A, Ayuso Colella JR. Colonografía por TC. Lo que el radiólogo debe conocer. Radiologia. 2011;53(4):315–25.

Introduction to Structured Reporting

3

Jacob J. Visser ⓘ
and Erik R. Ranschaert ⓘ

Contents

J. J. Visser (✉)
Department of Radiology & Nuclear Medicine, Erasmus MC,
Rotterdam, The Netherlands
e-mail: j.j.visser@erasmusmc.nl

E. R. Ranschaert
Department of Radiology, Elisabeth-TweeSteden Hospital (ETZ),
Tilburg, The Netherlands

Ghent University, Ghent, Belgium
e-mail: e.ranschaert@etz.nl

© European Society of Medical Imaging Informatics
(EuSoMII) 2022
M. Fatehi, D. Pinto dos Santos (eds.), *Structured Reporting in
Radiology*, Imaging Informatics for Healthcare Professionals,
https://doi.org/10.1007/978-3-030-91349-6_3

3.1   Introduction

Since radiology is a supporting specialty with a mainly consultative function, the radiological report is an essential part of the service rendered by radiologists to the referring clinicians and their patients. It is the core of the communication by the radiologist and in a way the product at the end stage of the workflow [1]. The basic purpose of reporting is unchanged from what it was a century ago. The value of the radiologist lies in his or her ability to recognize and coherently describe relevant findings, as well as to provide an opinion on the clinical implications. According to several papers, a radiology report is considered to be good if it is clear, correct, complete, and consistent and contains confidence level [2–4]. Unfortunately, today in most cases, the radiology report is still a piece of prose, consisting of a description of the findings followed by a problem-oriented interpretation of those findings.

Michael Porter introduced in 2006 the concept of value-based healthcare. Instead of looking at the volume for reimbursement, he urged to consider the added value of the care process as a base for reimbursement for healthcare providers [5]. In response to this, the American College of Radiology introduced a strategic initiative to introduce the concept of value-based healthcare in imaging. Boland addresses this topic in a series of articles in the Journal of the American College of Radiology [6, 7]. He mentioned that the key for radiologists to ensure value is to optimize the impact of the image interpretation reports.

The introduction of digital solutions such as PACS and RIS, together with speech recognition software, has significantly influenced the way of reporting and had a positive impact on the radiological workflow. It also brought new opportunities to improve the radiological report, not only by speeding up its availability but also by automatically adding relevant information to the report, such as clinical information and question definition. Partly thanks to these improvements, the long-standing demand for standardized and structured reporting is only getting stronger [1]. The increasing importance and value of radiologists in multidisciplinary decision-making in the treatment processes of patients and the gradual introduction of new technologies such as artificial intelligence (AI) probably also significantly affect this growing trend toward structured reporting.

3.2   What Is a Radiology Report?

One of the earliest known radiology reports is the letter written in 1896 by Dr. William J. Morton, in which he describes an abdominal radiograph [8]. Although the imaging methods changed radically with the introduction of new modalities like ultrasound, computed tomography, and magnetic resonance imaging, from this letter it appears that until today, within a period of more than a century, radiologists in general kept using narrative reports.

The radiology report is the essential work product of the diagnostic radiologists and represents the culmination of the radiologist's reading of a medical imaging study [8]. It is a formal document, representing the radiologist's official interpretation. It also shows largely how most radiologists conduct patient care, and it is the product by which clinicians gauge our value. It is the medium by which patients most frequently interact with radiologists, maybe their only interaction.

The basic components of the radiological report are explained in the Practice Guideline for Communication of the American College of Radiology (ACR) [9] and the Guidelines for Radiological Reporting of the European Society of Radiology (ESR) [10].

The report is the cornerstone of the communication between the radiologist and the referring physician. A typical report holds the clinical indication for the exam, a description of the findings, and a conclusion or impression. Each radiological examination must result in a final (official) written report, regardless of where the examination took place.

Although the radiology report may not immediately be seen as a subject related to imaging informatics, one should keep in mind that a large part of informatics is also related to information science. The radiology report is the way in which radiologists pass on the information they produce to others in order to care for the patient, which nowadays mostly happens in a digital format. This also means that a lot of information technology is involved in the way radiologists distribute this information.

In the past decade, there have been increasing efforts toward using structured reporting and lexicons to promote greater standardization, with the overall goal of improving radiologists' value through enhanced communications. With technology advancements such as speech recognition and AI, including Natural Language Processing (NLP), the reporting solutions are becoming more intelligent to enhance the workflow of the radiologists and to improve their work product.

3.3   Speech Recognition

For several decades, radiologists used tape recording to generate reports. Transcriptionists changed the verbally generated text into a written report that was approved by the reporting radiologist. With the introduction of speech recognition, transcriptionists were no longer needed. Instead, radiologists were able to immediately see the spoken text on the screen, and a written report was generated immediately. This also speeded up the availability of reports for referring physicians. Thanks to speech recognition, radiologists can report their findings almost in real time and send the result to the Radiology Information System (RIS) or the Electronic Health Record (EHR). Indispensable as speech recognition may be these days, it can also be the cause of many errors due to faulty pronunciation, accent, poor microphone position, background noise, the inability of the system to recognize particular words, etc. Speech engines are getting better, however, and a form of AI called natural language processing (NLP) is gradually being introduced [11]. NLP is capable of filtering meaningful information from dictation, from which it can automatically produce structured reports. It facilitates text and data search and thus can be used to automatically correct reports. Ideally, NLP would systematically screen reports for critical terms and warn the radiologist that urgent action needs to be undertaken [12].

3.4 Structure and Content of Structured Radiology Reports

The term, structured reporting, is commonly used in radiology. However, there is no set, agreed-upon definition of the term. Instead, it is used to describe various reporting techniques. Hence, the term has become confusing to some. Many have promoted structured reporting over free-text, prose-style reporting, but it is not without issues. Implementation of structured reporting is complex, with potentially a significant impact on radiologists' workflow.

According to Langlotz, there are three distinct attributes to a structured report: format, organization, and terminology [13].

- The format refers to the layout of the radiology report, which should be uniform.
- Consistent organization of the reports includes division of the text into separate sections with headings (e.g., "Findings" and "Conclusion"). Langlotz also advocates a consistent organization of the imaging observations, which has also been described as itemized or "template" reporting.
- Usage of standard terminology is the third attribute, which should avoid miscommunications caused by different interpretations of a report by referring providers.

These thoughts are also reflected in the ESR opinion paper on structured reporting in radiology. According to the ESR, a structured report should meet some basic elements in order to be useful for radiologists as well as for referring physicians. Some elements to consider are the following:

- The report should match the clinical question taking into account what is appropriate in the specific context.
- The report must be responsive to specific clinical circumstances.
- Medical procedures and clinical situations must be categorized.
- There should be a consensus among radiologists, referring physicians and societies about the elements of the report.

These basic elements need to be reflected in a structured format, a so-called "template", as also Langlotz refers to. For all these items, it needs to be mentioned that it is an iterative process requiring continuous monitoring and evaluation with subsequent adjustments [14].

When considering structured reporting, attention should also be paid to including staging systems (TNM, etc.), procedural components, complications, and even quantitative biomarker information.

3.5   Reasons for Structured Reporting

The most important reasons for implementing structured reporting are the need to improve the quality of the reports, the need for datafication and quantification of reporting elements, and to improve the accessibility of the reports. See also Fig. 3.1 for the benefits of structured reporting.

The quality of the report will be improved as standardization is introduced or increased. The aforementioned "template report" can serve as a checklist for particular examinations. Using such a list will ensure that information is provided that is relevant to the

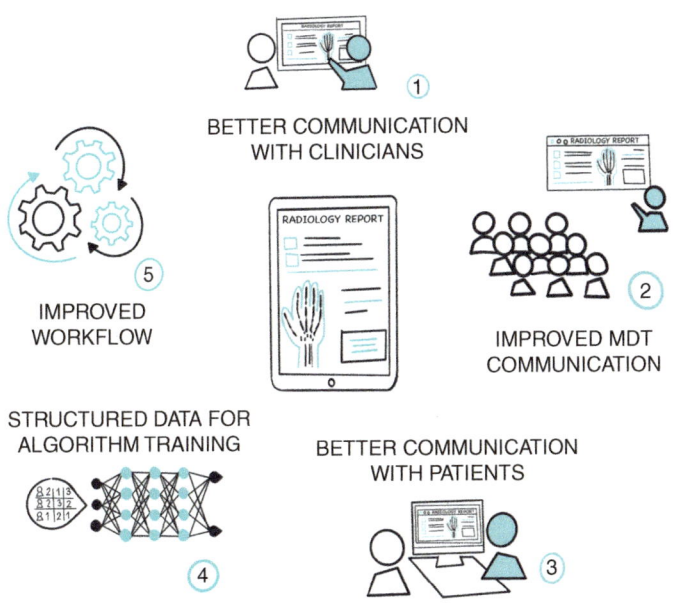

Fig. 3.1 Benefits of structured reporting

clinical question. Some of these items can be case dependent, such as the hippocampal volume in an MRI of the brain for a patient with dementia. Usage of standardized terminology facilitates the comparability of diseases and the evaluation of treatments. For specific examinations in oncology, several dedicated scoring systems are nowadays available, such as PI-RADS for prostate cancer and BI-RADS for breast cancer, which facilitate wide-scale implementation of standardized terminology [15]. Using standardized terminology prevents ambiguity and will provide greater guidance for determining the next steps in the diagnostic process and/or treatment decision. Having standardized reporting in place, the comparison of results will be easier.

In current clinical practice, free text reports may not sufficiently address the clinical question, which is increasingly asking for quantifiable information, especially in oncology. The report should include data elements and quantified imaging biomarkers, which also requires further integration of tools and systems that provide such information with the goal of automatically incorporating such data elements into the report.

Although not yet fully leveraged by many, structured reporting has the potential to use its data elements with quantified metrics to do the following [14]:

- To automate functions (e.g., Tumor, Node, Metastasis (TNM) staging, RECIST evaluation)
- To integrate with other data sources (e.g., radiomics, laboratory results, pathology findings)
- To share data with external entities (e.g., registries such as national cancer registries or biobanks)
- To perform data mining for research, education, quality improvement, and operational enhancements

As data is becoming increasingly relevant, it is of great importance to generate the interpretation of images in a standardized and structured way so that these interpretations can be used by other systems. By doing so, the information from the report can feed many clinical decisions. Also, the availability of this data allows for the evaluation of the quality and added value of radiology. Therefore, the data must be stored in a structured and standardized format allowing for easy access for relevant (third) parties.

3.6   Barriers to Structured Reporting

Although most radiologists agree on the advantage of structured reporting, significant barriers are present. These issues include the lack of standardization in reporting, the lack of technical support, and the scarcity of structured reporting-based software applications. And last but not least, radiologists are afraid that the introduction of structured reporting requires significant time investments and will slow down the workflow [11, 16].

3.7 Artificial Intelligence

For training of algorithms, the radiological report is often used as ground truth, usually in combination with other patient-related information such as clinical data and laboratory findings. For training solid medical imaging AI models, an accurate match between this data and the images is a prerequisite [17]. At present, however, the overwhelming majority of reports remain composed of free text. If radiology would be able to deliver structured data for all examinations, routine reports could be used for the development of artificial intelligence tools.

Following the existing guidelines for reporting diagnostic imaging aiming toward structured reporting would immensely reduce the effort needed to extract useful imaging labels. Novel semantic reporting systems that aim to index and codify free-text reports in real time are being developed but are currently not widely available yet [17].

3.8 Personalized Healthcare

In addition, as structured reporting requires predefined templates, it will be possible to include all relevant data in the report so that the referring physician can use this information in the personalized treatment of the patient. This will also increase the quality of the report.

3.9 Standard Terminology

Standard clinical terms, codes, and ontologies play an important role in improving clarity and interoperability [18]. In computer science and information science, an ontology is a set of concepts and the relationships between those concepts for a particular subject. For example, RadLex is an ontology focused on the subject of radiology.

Ideally, structured reports are related to an underlying nomenclature or ontology, such as SNOMED, LOINC, or Radlex. The use of these international standards also allows for automated translation of reports, extraction of data for scientific and epidemiologic purposes, and the possibility to feed machine and deep learning software.

To facilitate these efforts, international standards such as DICOM Structured Reporting (DICOM SR) should be used for structured reporting [19]. DICOM SR uses traditional DICOM messaging as well as DICOMweb.

The RSNA and ESR both support the MRRT (Management of Radiology Report Templates), which is the International Health Enterprise (IHE)'s integration profile dedicated to providing reporting templates. These templates are provided in a syntax enabling direct management through web browsers because MRRT uses Hypertext Transfer Protocol (HTTP) protocol. Using coded entries such as RadLex increases the accessibility of reports, as previously mentioned.

RadElement Common Data Elements (CDEs) are standardized sets of questions and allowable answers in radiology [20]. These elements are uniform and defined in a data dictionary. The name of the entity and its data type specifies the CDE. For example, for a lung nodule, a query may be "nodule diameter", which has an ID of RDE607, with the answer being a numerical value in mm units with a step value of 0.1. CDEs can enhance radiology reporting, data analysis, research, and decisions that support and improve data exchange. They are already in place for various domains such as cancer and stroke [21].

3.10 Availability of Templates

The Radiological Society of North America (RSNA) has developed a free online library of "best practices" reporting templates at radreport.org. Each template has been designed utilizing appropriate terminology (e.g., RadLex) and is based on best practices and established technical standards. Many of the RadReport templates are currently based on the IHE MRRT profile. CDEs can also be incorporated. In a joint effort to facilitate the usage of such templates on a wider scale, the RSNA and European Society of Radiology (ES) established the Template Library Advisory Panel (TLAP) [14]. The TLAP is responsible for the following:

- To provide expertise for the development of radiology reporting templates (clinical content and technical formatting)
- To solicit and develop reporting templates for inclusion in RSNA's report template library (www.RadReport.org)
- To review templates submitted by RSNA members and members of collaborating societies (e.g., ESR) to the template library
- To annotate report templates in the select library with terms from RadLex and other ontologies

3.11 The Future Radiology Report

The radiology report will remain the primary communication tool for the radiologist. However, the radiologists' focus should not be limited to the referring physician since also patients will increasingly obtain access to their reports. Structured reporting could facilitate these developments by potentially creating adapted versions of a report, namely a physician's version containing professional medical terms and a patient's version containing understandable language for the patient.

In addition, the future report will be rich in metadata allowing for several other functions including linking to other databases [11]. By doing so, structured reporting delivers data further downstream in the healthcare process.

For various conditions, the treatment of the disease is indicated in guidelines. The decisions made for an individual patient depend on the personal health profile and genetic data. If the data from the radiological report can automatically be included in these guidelines, this information can also be incorporated in the guidelines [11]. In this way, the data from the structured report can also be used as input for clinical decision support systems that enable personalized diagnosis and treatment plans.

3.12 Implementation

Although numerous surveys have shown that both radiologists and referring physicians prefer structured reports, the narrative report has undergone little or no change in the course of 120 years. Despite multiple advantages of structuring the radiology report, many radiologists are still reluctant to embrace the idea, which delays its large-scale introduction. To increase the adoption among radiologists, several issues need to be considered:

- Further standardization of terminology and lexicon
- Further acceptance of technical standards for structured reporting by vendors
- Seamless of software facilitating the radiological workflow
- Adaptation of speech recognition models offering hybrid solutions offering both structured reporting and self-editing modes
- Increasing the radiologists' awareness about the value of SR
- Increasing the collaboration between radiologists and referring physicians designing templates
- Education of radiology trainees or residents with structured reporting

It is important to gain experience with developing templates and using structured reporting in clinical practice. Once several successful pilots have been carried out and the results are published for the radiological community, adoption is highly likely to increase.

3.13 Education

During the training of radiology residents, little attention is paid to reporting skills. The ability to communicate radiological findings, either in a multidisciplinary context or individually to referring doctors and patients, should be considered an essential part of radiological training. In addition, it is also important that young radiologists gain insight into the possibilities of a digitally structured report, not only with regard to the underlying technical aspects, but also with regard to the possibilities of enriching these reports with other data, so that they can be reused for higher-level purposes, such as construction of decision support systems and AI algorithms.

It is currently possible to evaluate the reporting skills of radiology assistants through some digital platforms, but it is not yet part of their formal training. Most tests and evaluation programs primarily focus on the assessment skills of the residents rather than their ability to produce a coherent and correct radiological report [2].

Given the increasing importance of good communication in radiology and medicine, it is undoubtedly worthwhile to pay sufficient attention to the reporting skills of future radiologists, including teaching them in what ways structured reporting can add value to their role as radiologists. This of course also means that the necessary resources and infrastructure are made available for this and that the generation of established radiologists takes the lead in this.

References

1. Flanders AE, Lakhani P. Radiology reporting and communications: a look forward. Neuroimaging Clin N Am. 2012;22(3):477–96.
2. Wallis A, McCoubrie P. The radiology report—are we getting the message across? Clin Radiol. 2011;66(11):1015–22.
3. Friedman PJ. Radiologic reporting: structure. AJR Am J Roentgenol. 1983;140(1):171–2.
4. Hall FM. Language of the radiology report: primer for residents and wayward radiologists. AJR Am J Roentgenol. 2000;175(5):1239–42.
5. Porter ME. What is value in health care? N Engl J Med. 2010;363(26):2477–81.
6. Boland GW, Duszak R Jr. Structured reporting and communication. J Am Coll Radiol. 2015;12(12 Pt A):1286–8.
7. Boland GW, et al. Delivery of appropriateness, quality, safety, efficiency and patient satisfaction. J Am Coll Radiol. 2014;11(1):7–11.

8. Brady AP. Radiology reporting—from Hemingway to HAL? Insights Imaging. 2018;9(2):237–46.
9. Sherry CAM, Berlin L, Fajardo L, Gazelle G. ACR practice guideline for communicationof diagnostic imaging findings. 2011.
10. European Society of Radiology. Good practice for radiological reporting. Guidelines from the European Society of Radiology (ESR). Insights Imaging. 2011;2(2):93–6.
11. Ranschaert ER, Bosmans J. Report communication standards. Berlin Heidelberg: Springer; 2017.
12. Spandorfer A, et al. Deep learning to convert unstructured CT pulmonary angiography reports into structured reports. Eur Radiol Exp. 2019;3(1):37.
13. Langlotz CP. The radiology report: a guide to thoughtful communication for radiologists and other medical professionals. 2015.
14. European Society of Radiology. ESR paper on structured reporting in radiology. Insights Imaging. 2018;9(1):1–7.
15. Huicochea Castellanos S, Gonzalez-Aguirre A, Chapa Ibargüengoitia M, Vazquez SE, Vazquez Lamadrid J; Mexico, DF/MX, BI-RADS, C-RADS, GI-RADS, LI-RADS, Lu-RADS, TI-RADS, PI-RADS. The long and winding road of standardization, in ECR. Vienna; 2014.
16. Bosmans JM, et al. The radiology report as seen by radiologists and referring clinicians: results of the COVER and ROVER surveys. Radiology. 2011;259(1):184–95.
17. Willemink MJ, et al. Preparing medical imaging data for machine learning. Radiology. 2020;295(1):4–15.
18. Wang KC. Standard lexicons, coding systems and ontologies for interoperability and semantic computation in imaging. J Digit Imaging. 2018;31(3):353–60.
19. Hangiandreou NJ, Stekel SF, Tradup DJ. Comprehensive clinical implementation of DICOM structured reporting across a radiology ultrasound practice: lessons learned. J Am Coll Radiol. 2017;14(2):298–300.
20. Rubin DL, Kahn CE Jr. Common data elements in radiology. Radiology. 2017;283(3):837–44.
21. Toga AW, Dinov ID. Sharing big biomedical data. J Big Data. 2015;2:7.

Technical Considerations and Interoperable Reporting Standards

4

Peter Mildenberger, Mansoor Fatehi, and Daniel Pinto dos Santos

Contents

P. Mildenberger (✉)
Department of Radiology, University Medical Center Mainz, Mainz, Germany
e-mail: mildenbe@uni-mainz.de

M. Fatehi
Biobank, National Brain Mapping Laboratory, Tehran, Iran

D. Pinto dos Santos
Department of Radiology, University Hospital of Cologne, Cologne, Germany

© European Society of Medical Imaging Informatics (EuSoMII) 2022
M. Fatehi, D. Pinto dos Santos (eds.), *Structured Reporting in Radiology*, Imaging Informatics for Healthcare Professionals, https://doi.org/10.1007/978-3-030-91349-6_4

4.1   Introduction

Since the very early days of radiological reporting, the written radiological report is the most important contribution of the radiologist to patient management and care. Even though much has changed in radiology from a technical perspective since the late nineteenth century, especially with the introduction of a fully digitized workflow, the radiological report has basically remained unchanged and is mostly composed as some form of a letter from one physician to another [1].

While in its current form the traditional narrative radiological report certainly has some benefits in terms of efficiency and freedom to express all possible diagnostic findings, this format undoubtedly has some inherent downsides e.g., when it comes to automated extraction of information. Making the data contained in a radiological report accessible for further analysis could open up a new dimension for radiology as a specialty. One way to achieve this could be through the usage of pre-defined structured report templates, together with corresponding software tools that allow for the content of such structured reports to be accessed or shared with other software applications. Numerous use cases can be thought of, where such reusing of information from radiological reports could help streamline workflows or support efficient research—as Bosmans and co-authors rightly put it "Structured reporting: a fusion reactor hungry for fuel" [2]. Unsurprisingly, all major radiological societies have published statements highlighting the importance of the more widespread introduction of structured reporting into a clinical routine [3, 4].

It is, however, important to note here that the optimal solution is yet to be found. While some argue providing radiologists with various predefined and fixed report templates, each of which addresses a specific clinical scenario, others argue that a more flexible approach should be taken. Instead, radiologists could be provided with smaller report modules or elements, which could then be combined at the radiologists' discretion to compose the report needed to address the patient's specific situation.

Various interoperability standards have been proposed in the context of radiological reporting. In the DICOM standard, a corresponding object for structured reporting has existed for more than 20 years. In addition, the so-called clinical data architecture (CDA) by HL7 is important for encoding and transmitting clinical documents [5, 6]. For more detailed coding of specific findings, ontologies and terminologies such as RadLex, LOINC, and SNOMED are available. To establish an interoperable standard for structured reporting templates, integrating the healthcare enterprise (IHE) published the management of the radiology reporting template (MRRT) profile [7, 8]. More recently, the RSNA introduced the concept of common data elements (CDE) as a way to allow for more flexibility when constructing reporting templates while also ensuring comparable content [9].

4.2   How Much Structure Is Enough?

When we look at the history of structured reporting, it is interesting to note that proponents of the idea suggested its benefits as early as the 1920s. One of the earliest to advocate a more structured approach to radiology reporting was Preston Hickey, a radiologist from Detroit [10]. He noticed that due to their variability in language and style conventional narrative reports did not lend themselves to further analysis and therefore proposed standardized and structured report templates for radiographies. Now, one might ask, why is it that such structured forms of reporting radiological studies have failed to become the standard of practice in radiology?

One of the many relevant factors certainly is that no consensus exists as to what the optimal extent of structure in a radiological report is. With the introduction of fully digitized workflows in radiology, it may have seemed obvious that computer software allowing for detailed structuring of radiology reports would soon become the go-to solution—especially given that many radiologists in the early days were not particularly fond of speech recognition [11]. However, it soon became clear that among other

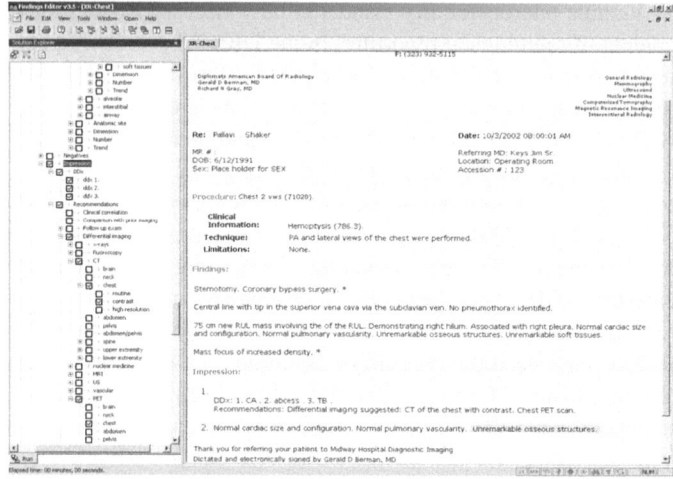

Fig. 4.1 Example of an early software for structured reporting (StructuRad)

factors many of the proposed systems would overwhelm the radiologists with too detailed structuring of findings (Fig. 4.1).

Unlike some other professions where implementation of such systems may have been the obvious choice, radiology and healthcare in general pose specific challenges when thinking about changes in workflow. Radiologists' workload is steadily increasing; e.g., the relative value units (RVUs) per year and full-time equivalent (FTE) radiologist have increased by around 70% in the time between 1991 and 2007 [12]. From these numbers alone, it is quite clear that any change in the workflow that slows the reporting process rather than speeding it up will be difficult to implement. For structured reporting to be adopted in clinical routine, it will therefore be essential to think about what information really needs to be structured and which parts of the report can be left in the form of narrative text. This may not always be easy to determine, but the following considerations might help to guide future developments here.

Just as the clinical scenarios in which imaging is needed can differ widely, so does the potential—and in fact the need—for structuring the radiological report vary. Cases such as CT for acute abdominal pain in a complex postoperative abdomen are obviously not ideal for structured reporting. There are innumerable potential causes depending on what surgery has been performed earlier. Providing a structure to capture all possibilities would be almost impossible, or at the very least would make for an incredibly complex report template that would be difficult to navigate. On the other hand, many routine cases would greatly benefit from structured reports. This can be nicely exemplified for the case of primary CT staging for pancreatic ductal adenocarcinoma (PDAC). According to the guidelines published by the National Comprehensive Cancer Network (NCCN), the potential respectability of the tumor can be determined by imaging and largely depends on the vascular involvement of the tumor (Fig. 4.2) [13, 14]. However, not every individual radiologist may be aware of what information is relevant to the surgeon, especially in subspecialized environments. Of course, the expert on radiological assessment of PDAC will be familiar with the relevant report items, but when he or she is unavailable, someone else will need to report the case. Various studies have shown that report templates tailored to a specific pathology (in this case, PDAC) ensure that relevant information is included in the reports, which would have been missing in conventional narrative reports [15, 16].

Whenever thinking about structured reporting, it should be important to keep the above said in mind. The ultimate goal could in theory be to structure every part of the report, so that all information is available for detailed further analysis. However, in the foreseeable future, it is somewhat unlikely that an easy-to-use method of structuring the complete report can be found that does

PRINCIPLES OF DIAGNOSIS, IMAGING, AND STAGING
PANCREATIC CANCER RADIOLOGY REPORTING TEMPLATE[1]

Arterial Evaluation				
SMA Contact	☐ Present	☐ Absent		
Degree of solid soft-tissue contact	☐ ≤180	☐ >180		
Degree of increased hazy attenuation/ stranding contact	☐ ≤180	☐ >180		
Focal vessel narrowing or contour irregularity	☐ Present	☐ Absent		
Extension to first SMA branch	☐ Present	☐ Absent		

Fig. 4.2 Excerpt of the NCCN report template for PDAC [13]

not negatively impact the radiologist's workflow. Large parts of a report could be left unstructured as free text, as long as those parts that are relevant to guide clinical decision-making in a specific scenario (e.g., PDAC, see above) are contained in a corresponding structured report template. Such an approach would ensure high-quality radiological reports, while leaving enough room to describe normal and abnormal findings at the radiologist's discretion that would be difficult to capture in a structured form.

4.3 Structured Data Entry or Structured Content Output?

All of the above implies that the main way to structure report data should be structured data entry into a respective reporting system (of which currently there is only a limited number). Also, when looking at the NCCN template (Fig. 4.2), one could argue that such a tabular presentation of findings might be helpful during the reporting process, but less optimal as a format to present the report to the referring physician or patient. This leads to two important questions that sometimes are forgotten when talking about structured reporting. Do we really need to force radiologists to use a structured report data entry system and what is the most desirable report output format?

Interestingly, there have been only a few studies addressing the latter question. From what is available in the scientific literature, it seems that the information contained in a report can be transferred to the reader equally well irrespective of the format [17]. However, when asking referring physicians about their subjective preference, most tend to prefer a tabular format with "telegraphic" constructions such as "Liver: normal" [18–20].

Certainly, when using a structured data input format, getting the desired output format is easily done. In order to get a structured output, little work is needed since potentially the tabular format in which the data has been input can just be used as is. To get a seemingly less-structured output resembling a free narrative report, the only steps needed are to assign sentences and modifiers to any given combination of structured inputs. This can easily be done and in fact is the solution most vendors of structured reporting software offer today (Fig. 4.3).

In contrast, the other way around (i.e., converting initially unstructured reports to structured data) is technically much more challenging, albeit in many cases highly desirable. Most importantly, such techniques to convert could open up interesting opportunities to retrospectively analyze the large amount of report data that has been collected in radiological departments to this day. But in cases where providing a structured data input form would be impractical due to a large number of possible options (e.g., in cases CT for acute abdomen in a postoperative setting, see above), such methods could allow to consistently provide referring physicians with structured and tabular reports. To achieve this goal, some form of natural language processing (NLP) will be needed. In fact, over the last years, many studies have been published generally showing good to very good per-

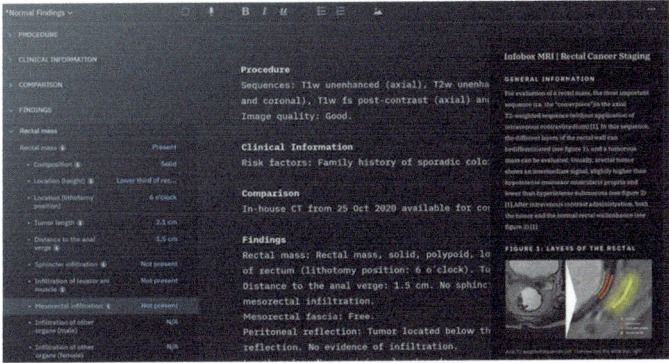

Fig. 4.3 Example of a structured reporting software (Smart Reporting, Munich, Germany). The software produces a seemingly free narrative report text based on a structured data input

formance—although in some instances limited to specific use cases [21]. Nevertheless, two major drawbacks must be mentioned when considering the usage of NLP on narrative radiological reports. First, and most obviously, any NLP algorithm can only extract and structure information that is present in the original report in the first place. As mentioned earlier, e.g., for preoperative assessment of PDAC, this is not always the case and largely depends on the radiologist's experience [15]. Second, despite the NLP algorithms in most cases capturing the information provided in the narrative texts accurately, there may be instances in which the intended meaning of parts of the report are inadvertently changed. For example, in a Dutch study out of 22 T1-stage lung cancers, the NLP algorithm misclassified two as being T3 and one as being T4 [22]. Conversely, out of 30 T4-stage tumors, two ended up being classified as T2 and one as T1. It is easy to see how this could negatively impact the respective patient's management if the result of the NLP algorithm is not thoroughly checked before providing the resulting report document to the referring physician. Among other factors, this might be one that explains why NLP has not yet made its way to clinical routine and is mainly only used in research settings [21].

There may, however, also be a third option—hybrid reporting. In its most simple form, only those pieces of information that are relatively easy and safe to extract from reports, like measurements of sizes together with their descriptors, are extracted and output in a structured format [23]. Coming back to the example in PDAC assessment mentioned previously, in which only the relevant information is structured in a corresponding report template at the input level, another hybrid approach seems promising, too. In this case, any additional information that is provided as free text could potentially be structured using NLP [24] (Fig. 4.4). Such an approach would combine the potential benefits of structured report templates (high report quality by ensuring all relevant information is contained), while also providing means to make unstructured data accessible and at the same time mitigating the

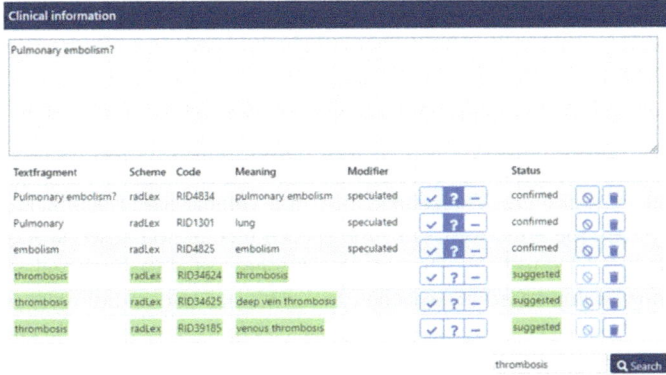

Fig. 4.4 Example of a software solution using hybrid reporting (MRRE; Jungmann et al.)

risk that information crucial to the particular situation of the patient could inadvertently be misclassified.

4.4   Speech Recognition and Structured Reporting

Speech recognition in radiology report creation has quite a long history already. In 1987, one of the first systems to be successfully introduced into clinical practice was presented by Kurzweil Applied Intelligence [25]. It was able to recognize around words from a lexicon comprising around 1000 entries. However, due to technical limitations, mainly in computational power, composing a radiological report using this technology took 20% longer than dictating it and having it transcribed by a human. Since then, much has improved and speech recognition has become the standard in most institutions [26].

Compared to most currently available structured reporting solutions, speech recognition offers one key advantage—it is incredibly fast and convenient. It allows the radiologist to keep the mouse pointer on the images for the most part of the reporting process, hence enabling interactions like changing window/level settings and performing measurements, while simultaneously allowing for the report to be composed. Compared to that, many currently available "point-and-click" structured reporting systems require the user to move the mouse pointer across the screen to interact with the report and then back to the image to continue interaction there. Understandably, in a volume-based healthcare system, the effectiveness of the speech-recognition-based workflow is hard to beat. This might, of course, change if and when more value-based approaches to healthcare and radiology are implemented—or at least if usage of structured reporting is incentivized by the relevant authorities through conditioning reimbursement on it [27, 28].

On the other hand, both approaches could potentially be combined to form what some authors call the "perfect reporting system" [29]. Creating such software would certainly be no easy feat. Most importantly, the system would have to be able to correctly understand any type and combination of words and sentences with identical meaning, including possible ambiguities, and translate the information into the respective structured data format. Nonetheless, such an ideal system could still guide the reporting process by offering speech-enabled navigation through the report template, thereby leveraging the value of report templates to ensure report quality and completeness while allowing the reporting radiologist to keep the mouse pointer on the images for uninterrupted interaction.

Over the last years, some remarkable technological advances have been made so that the development of such systems might seem more achievable than ever. And the advantages of combining speech recognition with structured reporting templates seem so obvious that vendors have already started to present first implementations of such systems. However, in most cases, the system does not allow for completely unrestricted speech input. Nonetheless, speech-enabled interaction with the report templates might just be the one key component that has been missing to allow for smooth integration of structured reporting into the radiological routine workflow.

4.5   DICOM Structured Reporting

Whatever the workflow to produce structured reports may be in the future, solutions will be needed to allow for interoperable technical representations of the radiological report. One of the first standards aiming to define how clinical observations related to medical imaging should be structured was the DICOM Structured Reporting (SR) object. In principle, DICOM SR objects are intended to support image-based diagnostics or intervention in the acquisition of specific data, which may be reference images, measurements, ROI, radiation exposure data, etc. Thus, the use of DICOM SR objects plays its actual role in the stage before the actual report generation. The advantage of the concept of DICOM is the integration into the existing PACS infrastructure and the DICOM communication processes between different modalities and IT systems. DICOM SR objects can be created at various points or process steps. Examples include the creation of DICOM Radiation Dose SR directly at the examination modality in order to transmit the radiation exposure to central systems for the acquisition and analysis of dose values. Other applications arise, for example, in the measurement of velocity values in duplex sonography. Here, DICOM SR objects can be used to transfer a set of measured values directly to a reporting system, thus avoiding manual input in the reporting process and minimizing workload and sources of error. It can also be used in postprocessing, in which computer-based evaluations are documented in a structured manner at a corresponding workstation, stored using appropriate DICOM SR templates, and then transferred to the further reporting process. DICOM-SR is therefore more of a supportive tool than a reporting system itself.

DICOM SR provides a great amount of flexibility; the DICOM standard does not impose any specific applications or input techniques for this purpose. DICOM-SR can therefore support the implementation of structured data acquisition in general. DICOM-SR documents adhere to the usual ways of encoding data elements in DICOM format as well as standard exchange procedures within a network (storage, query/retrieve).

Data structure follows the Patient-Study-Series model, and a hierarchical tree of "Content Items" is added. The captured information should be comprehensively defined by appropriate vocabularies or coding systems. These can be sources outside DICOM itself, such as LOINC, SNOMED, or RadLex. Within a DICOM SR template, the relationships between the various pieces of information are defined, typically in a parent–child structure that represents the relationships between the various pieces of information. The content itself may be represented as text, numeric values, codes, references to individual images or spatial coordinates, etc.

However, this flexibility can prove challenging, and systems that are to read these documents must be able to deal with the flexible structures in order to be able to analyze and display the structure and content correctly. To ensure comparability in terms of content across institutions and systems, according to the DICOM IODs, attributes can also be defined for DICOM SR templates, e.g., to specify which content is mandatory or optional [5, 6].

4.6   IHE Management of Radiology Reporting Templates (MRRT)

As DICOM SR did not seem optimal to develop and share templates for structured reporting, another representation of the medical information contained in radiological reports had to be found. While the RSNA's reporting initiative initially set for an XML-based scheme, this was later replaced by the HTML5-derived format suggested in the IHE MRRT profile [4, 7, 8].

This IHE profile addresses three different tasks:

- The creation of report templates (report template creator)
- The application of existing reporting templates (report creator)
- The provision of standardized reporting templates in a registry (report template manager)

As opposed to the more technical considerations that led to DICOM SR, the MRRT profile focuses more on the reporting process itself, where the three actors mentioned above support the workflow (Fig. 4.5). In addition, the transactions between the various actors are defined.

The three actors of the profile can be implemented and used separately, in combination or all at the same time in one reporting system. In principle, a radiological information system (RIS) can be limited to the use of existing templates. The profile defines how

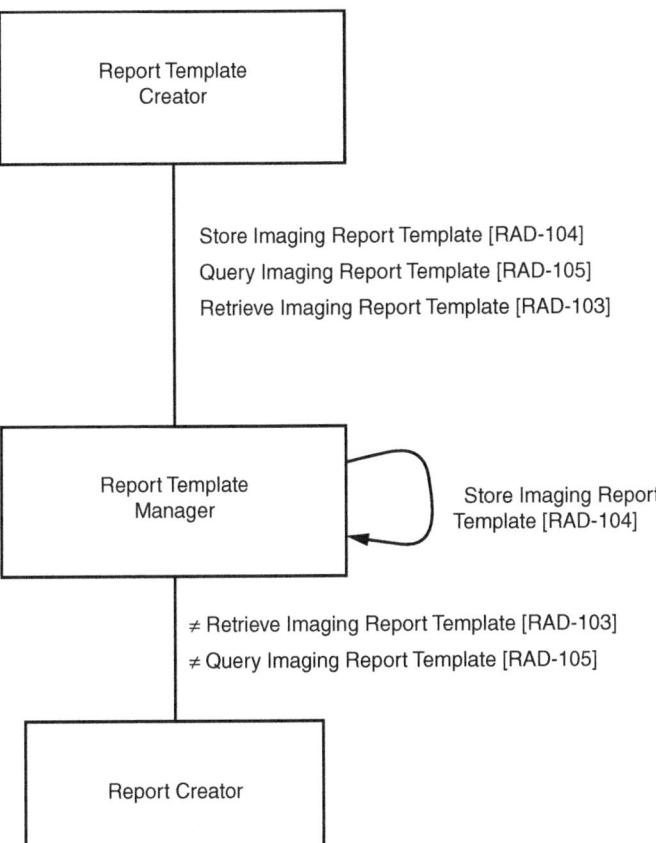

Fig. 4.5 MRRT actor diagram (IHE MRRT Profile V1.7, July 2018, Copyright by IHE International)

templates can be loaded from a repository and then used for reporting. Such collections of reporting templates are, e.g., provided in the Reporting Library (www.radreport.org) initiated by the RSNA. This has been a joint initiative of RSNA and ESR for several years now, with the Template Library Advisory Panel (TLAP) for review and approval of templates. Templates are available in different languages, and some templates have been developed in a consensus process by professional societies and thus in principle could have the highest priority with regard to common use in different institutions [30].

Template development can be done either with standard HTML code creation tools or with dedicated, freely available open-source solutions (T-Rex Report Template Editor, Vital Images). The interoperable MRRT format allows for templates to be used across RIS applications from different vendors while ensuring the same content is present in all instances. This means that in the reporting process itself, the sequence of content on which comments should be made is predefined and does not have to be recreated each time.

The MRRT profile describes specifications for the technical structure of the report templates. This includes the structure of the metadata as well as the individual content of a template and how contents should be coded. Individual fields of a template can represent different data types, and these can be clearly structured and categorized into descriptions of anatomy, localization, pathology, and so on. Common HTML data types like numerical values, text fields, and drop-down selection lists and checkboxes are permitted (Fig. 4.6).

An IHE MRI-based template primarily describes the content for a dedicated examination; the scope can be very wide, e.g., CT abdomen, or focused on a specific clinical question, e.g., pulmonary embolism. The implementation of the content and the way in which the radiologist works with such templates in the reporting process is left to the respective RIS. Due to the standardized transactions, a DICOM SR object, for example, with measured values from an ultrasound examination, can also be easily integrated into such report templates and thus the contents of a report can be automatically pre-filled. This significantly reduces manual interaction and sources of error.

Field Type	HTML5 Element	HTML5 Attribute	HTML5 Attribute Value
TEXT	input	type	text
TEXTAREA	textarea	-	-
NUMBER	input	type	number
SELECTION_LIST	select	multiple	single, multiple
DATE	input	type	date
TIME	input	type	time
CHECKBOX	input	type	checkbox
RADIO BUTTON	input	type	radio

Fig. 4.6 Attributes of report template fields (IHE MRRT Profile V1.7, July 2018, Copyright by IHE International)

There are various implementations within the scope of this IHE profile, for example, as an open-source web-based reporting platform that includes both the role of Report Template Manager and Report Creator [24, 31]. Such a solution can also be used additively to a RIS and integrated into the respective reporting process. The storage of template-based findings in a database then makes it possible to easily analyze report data on a large scale or use the data for secondary applications [32, 33]. This could prove especially useful in cross-institutional data collections, which could enable scientific evaluations in a very simple form.

4.7   Outlook

For further development of the standardization process in the field of structured reporting, an essential step is to achieve acceptance by users and manufacturers. Currently, the IHE MRRT profile still only has the status of trial implementation. However, the first steps have been made within the IHE Radiology Committee to finalize it. Another essential aspect is the acceptance and standardization of coding systems such as RadLex and SNOMED; until now, these have often been driven by billing processes and implemented less with regard to possible further scientific evaluation.

Over the last decade, various scientific societies have published position statements with clear recommendation for more widespread usage of structured reporting. It can be hoped that with recent technical advancements in incorporation of speech recognition and voice control into software products for structured reporting, a more user-friendly experience can be provided to radiologists that feel structured reporting interferes with their usual workflow and limits their productivity. Steps in the right direction have been made, and now it is time to start up the "fusion reactor hungry for fuel" [2].

References

1. Langlotz CP. The radiology report. Stanford; 2015.
2. Bosmans JML, Neri E, Ratib O, Kahn CE. Structured reporting: a fusion reactor hungry for fuel. Insights Imaging. 2015;6(1):129–32.
3. European Society of Radiology (ESR). ESR paper on structured reporting in radiology. Insights Imaging. 2018;9(1):1–7.
4. Morgan TA, Helibrun ME, Kahn CE. Reporting initiative of the Radiological Society of North America: progress and new directions. Radiology. 2014;273(3):642–5.
5. Noumeir R. Benefits of the DICOM structured report. J Digit Imaging. 2006;19(4):295–306.
6. Clunie D. DICOM structured reporting. PixelMed Publishing; 2000.
7. IHE Radiology Technical Committee, Herausgeber. IHE Radiology (RAD) White Paper—Management of Radiology Report Templates (MRRT). 2012.
8. IHE Radiology Technical Committee. IHE Radiology Technical Framework Supplement—Management of Radiology Report Templates (MRRT). 2018.
9. Rubin DL, Kahn CE. Common data elements in radiology. Radiology. 2017;283(3):837–44.
10. Hickey P. Standardization of Roentgen-ray reports. Am J Roentgenol. 1922;9:422–5.
11. Langlotz CP. Enhancing the expressiveness of structured reporting systems. J Digit Imaging. 2000;13(S1):49–53.
12. Bhargavan M, Kaye AH, Forman HP, Sunshine JH. Workload of radiologists in United States in 2006–2007 and trends since 1991–1992. Radiology. 2009;252(2):458–67.
13. Tempero MA, Malafa MP, Al-Hawary M, Asbun H, Bain A, Behrman SW, u. a. Pancreatic adenocarcinoma, version 2.2017, NCCN clinical

practice guidelines in oncology. J Natl Compr Cancer Netw. 2017;15(8):1028–61.

14. Hong SB, Lee SS, Kim JH, Kim HJ, Byun JH, Hong SM, u. a. Pancreatic cancer CT: prediction of resectability according to NCCN criteria. Radiology. 2018;289(3):710–8.

15. Brook OR, Brook A, Vollmer CM, Kent TS, Sanchez N, Pedrosa I. Structured reporting of multiphasic CT for pancreatic cancer: potential effect on staging and surgical planning. Radiology. 2015;274(2):464–72.

16. Dimarco M, Cannella R, Pellegrino S, Iadicola D, Tutino R, Allegra F, u. a. Impact of structured report on the quality of preoperative CT staging of pancreatic ductal adenocarcinoma: assessment of intra- and inter-reader variability. Abdom Radiol. 2020;45(2):437–48.

17. Sistrom CL, Honeyman-Buck J. Free text versus structured format: information transfer efficiency of radiology reports. Am J Roentgenol. 2005;185(3):804–12.

18. Plumb AAO, Grieve FM, Khan SH. Survey of hospital clinicians' preferences regarding the format of radiology reports. Clin Radiol. 2009;64(4):386–94.

19. Camilo DMR, Tibana TK, Adôrno IF, Santos RFT, Klaesener C, Gutierrez Junior W, et al. Radiology report format preferred by requesting physicians: prospective analysis in a population of physicians at a university hospital. Radiol Bras. 2019;52(2):97–103.

20. Bosmans JML, Weyler JJ, De Schepper AM, Parizel PM. The radiology report as seen by radiologists and referring clinicians: results of the COVER and ROVER surveys. Radiology. 2011;259(1):184–95.

21. Pons E, Braun LMM, Hunink MGM, Kors JA. Natural language processing in radiology: a systematic review. Radiology. 2016;279(2):329–43.

22. Nobel JM, Puts S, Bakers FCH, Robben SGF, Dekker ALAJ. Natural language processing in Dutch free text radiology reports: challenges in a small language area staging pulmonary oncology. J Digit Imaging. 2020. http://link.springer.com/10.1007/s10278-020-00327-z.

23. Bozkurt S, Alkim E, Banerjee I, Rubin DL. Automated detection of measurements and their descriptors in radiology reports using a hybrid natural language processing algorithm. J Digit Imaging. 2019;32(4):544–53.

24. Jungmann F. A hybrid reporting platform for extended RadLex coding combining structured reporting templates and natural language processing. J Digit Imaging. 2020;33(4):1026–33.

25. Robbins A, Horowitz D, Srinivasan M, Vincent M, Shaffer K, Sadowsky N, et al. Speech-controlled generation of radiology reports. Radiology. 1987;164(2):569–73.

26. Hammana I, Lepanto L, Poder T, Bellemare C, Ly M-S. Speech recognition in the radiology department: a systematic review. Health Inf Manag J. 2015;44(2):4–10.

27. Brady AP, Bello JA, Derchi LE, Fuchsjäger M, Goergen S, Krestin GP, et al. Radiology in the era of value-based healthcare: a multi-society

expert statement from the ACR, CAR, ESR, IS3R, RANZCR, and RSNA. Insights Imaging. 2020;11(1):136.

28. Goldberg-Stein S, Chernyak V. Adding value in radiology reporting. J Am Coll Radiol. 2019;16(9):1292–8.

29. Liu D, Zucherman M, Tulloss WB. Six characteristics of effective structured reporting and the inevitable integration with speech recognition. J Digit Imaging. 2006;19(1):98–104.

30. Pinto dos Santos D, Hempel J-M, Mildenberger P, Klöckner R, Persigehl T. Structured reporting in clinical routine. RöFo - Fortschritte Auf Dem Geb Röntgenstrahlen Bildgeb Verfahr. 2019;191(01):33–9.

31. Pinto dos Santos D, Klos G, Kloeckner R, Oberle R, Dueber C, Mildenberger P. Development of an IHE MRRT-compliant open-source web-based reporting platform. Eur Radiol. 2017;27(1):424–30.

32. Pinto dos Santos D, Scheibl S, Arnhold G, Maehringer-Kunz A, Düber C, Mildenberger P, u. a. A proof of concept for epidemiological research using structured reporting with pulmonary embolism as a use case. Br J Radiol. 2018;91:20170564.

33. Pinto dos Santos D, Brodehl S, Baeßler B, Arnhold G, Dratsch T, Chon S-H, u. a. Structured report data can be used to develop deep learning algorithms: a proof of concept in ankle radiographs. Insights Imaging. 2019;10(1):93.

Template-Based Structured Reporting

5

Francesca Coppola
and Lorenzo Faggioni

Contents

F. Coppola (✉)
Malpighi Radiology Unit, S. Orsola Malpighi University Hospital,
Bologna, Italy
e-mail: francesca.coppola@aosp.bo.it

L. Faggioni
Diagnostic and Interventional Radiology, University Hospital of Pisa,
Pisa, Italy
e-mail: lfaggioni@sirm.org

© European Society of Medical Imaging Informatics
(EuSoMII) 2022
M. Fatehi, D. Pinto dos Santos (eds.), *Structured Reporting in
Radiology*, Imaging Informatics for Healthcare Professionals,
https://doi.org/10.1007/978-3-030-91349-6_5

5.1   Introduction

The radiological report is a fundamental step of radiologists' professional activity, by which the results and interpretation of a radiological procedure are formally documented in relation to the patient's history and clinical query [1]. Therefore, radiological reports should be prepared following criteria of completeness, clarity, and methodological rigor as prerequisites for an optimal communication with colleagues and patients.

Traditionally, radiological reports have been written using a narrative style based on free text language. Narrative reporting is deeply rooted in radiology history, as it is a simple and technically straightforward reporting method that does not require any complex IT infrastructure and grants unlimited freedom of expression to the reporting radiologist. However, too much content and style variability may involve the risk of composing unclear, incomplete, and/or inaccurate reports, thereby hindering its communicative effectiveness and overall clinical usefulness. Furthermore, advancements in medical knowledge and the growing availability of state-of-the-art technological equipment in radiology departments have broadened the spectrum of clinical indications to imaging (with particular reference to multidetector CT and MRI), opening up the opportunity to quickly obtain vast amounts of information that must be effectively summarized in radiological reports. In parallel, the development of validated recommendations and guidelines for the diagnostic and therapeutic management of several diseases calls for a more standardized reporting approach, taking into account all required information for a correct categorization of each individual patient's condition [2–4].

Structured reporting (SR) has the potential to overcome the limitations of narrative reporting, owing to its being based on a predefined digital "structure" that can be selected and at least partially modified at the user's discretion. From a practical viewpoint, standardized models (so-called templates) can be used for reporting that are user-selected based on the clinical setting and contain predefined types of information, such as alphanumeric data, free text, key images, movies, web links, and so on [5–8] (Fig. 5.1).

Major scientific societies have undertaken initiatives aimed to promote a widespread dissemination of radiological template-based SR, including the creation of standardized templates by RSNA, the joint RSNA/ESR initiative to translate RSNA templates into European languages, and the ESR paper on SR [9–14]. Unfortunately, so far such efforts have been faced with significant hurdles. A survey launched by the Imaging Informatics Chapter of the Italian Society of Medical and Interventional Radiology (SIRM) has shown that although most SIRM radiologist members

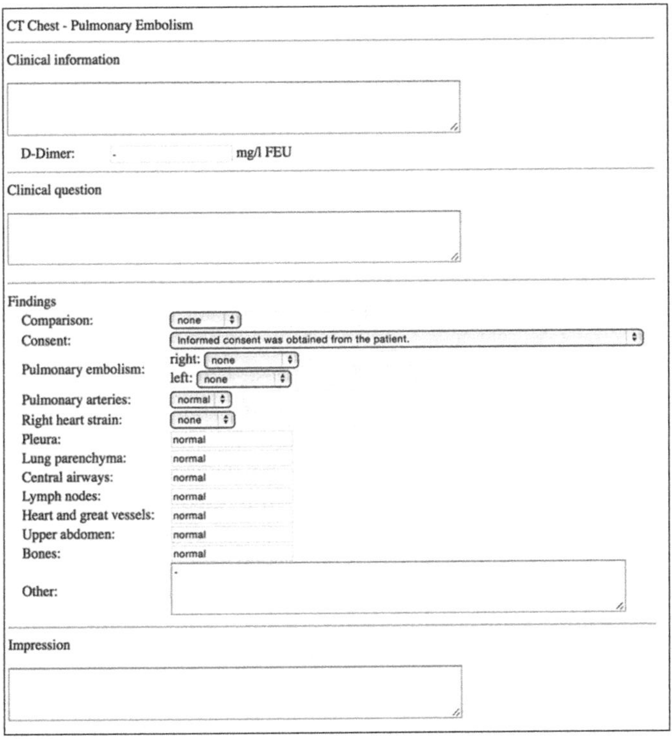
CT Chest - Pulmonary Embolism

Clinical information

D-Dimer: - mg/l FEU

Clinical question

Findings

Comparison: none

Consent: Informed consent was obtained from the patient.

Pulmonary embolism: right: none left: none

Pulmonary arteries: normal

Right heart strain: none

Pleura: normal

Lung parenchyma: normal

Central airways: normal

Lymph nodes: normal

Heart and great vessels: normal

Upper abdomen: normal

Bones: normal

Other: -

Impression

Fig. 5.1 Example of SR template for chest CT examinations performed in patients with suspected pulmonary embolism. Reproduced from [23] under a Creative Commons Attribution 4.0 International license (CC BY 4.0, http://creativecommons.org/licenses/by/4.0/)

were interested in SR and open to the possibility of using it, they were concerned that its adoption in their real working life could lead to semantic (i.e., definition, standardization, and validation of templates), technical (SR implementation and integration with existing RIS/PACS platforms), and professional issues (perception of the radiologist's professional role by other specialists and patients) [4].

In this chapter, the main pros and cons of template-based radiological SR versus narrative reporting will be discussed. Some hints will also be provided for a successful implementation of template-based SR in radiology practice.

5.2 Advantages of Template-Based SR over Narrative Reporting

The main strengths of template-based SR over narrative reporting include the following:

- *Standardized structure and terminology.* Standardized terminology is pivotal for adherence to diagnostic and/or therapeutic recommendations and enrolment in clinical trials [15], reduces the ambiguity that may arise from nonconventional language, and enables faster and more effective communication with other radiologists and nonradiologists [16–20]. Moreover, lexicon standardization and data categorization can favor trainees' learning [21, 22], aid reimbursement policies, and ease data mining and the creation of large multicenter databases (also called "big data") driving biomedical research, the development of guidelines, quality assurance processes, and epidemiological statistics [7, 23–25] (Fig. 5.2). Moreover, specific templates can be used that have been developed from evidence-based recommendations [20, 24]. Well-known examples of classification systems that naturally lend themselves to SR integration are the Reporting and Data Systems of the American College of Radiology; those include, e.g.,

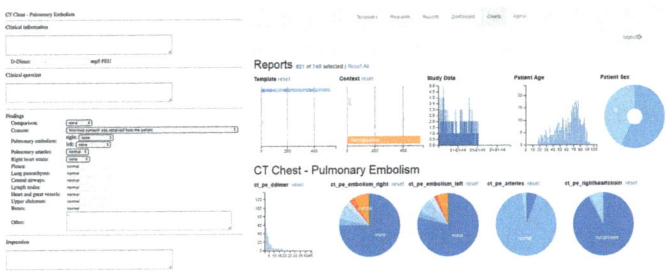

Fig. 5.2 Dashboard of summary results of all SR reports created with the SR template shown in Fig. 5.1, including patient's age and gender, D-dimer level, location of emboli, and signs of right heart failure. Reproduced from [23] under a Creative Commons Attribution 4.0 International license (CC BY 4.0, http://creativecommons.org/licenses/by/4.0/)

BI-RADS for breast imaging, LI-RADS for CT and MR imaging of hepatocellular carcinoma, LUNG-RADS for CT screening of lung cancer, or CAD-RADS for CT coronary angiography [25].

- *Key images and data-rich reports*. Template-based SR allows producing reports with a virtually unlimited information density ("data-rich") relatively quickly. In particular, the possibility to link images or other data to the report makes for clearer, more reproducible and easier-to-use reports, either for nonradiologists or other radiologists who may need to reassess a patient's case or report a follow-up examination of the same patient. For instance, it is possible to link key images or other data elements within a template-based SR that show the main findings of an imaging examination, resulting in improved communication [7, 8, 11, 19].
- *Better communication and greater clinical impact*. Various studies have shown that both radiologists and nonradiologists tend to prefer template-based SR to narrative reporting thanks to its greater effectiveness and clarity [17, 18, 26–32]. Such qualities can be especially appreciated in specific tasks of

higher complexity, owing to the greater ease of finding all necessary information for patient management. One of the areas that could benefit most from these characteristics is oncological imaging, due to the need to perform a systematic, accurate, and reproducible comparison of imaging findings at precise time frames of a patient's radiological history based on validated methods for treatment response assessment (e.g., RECIST criteria) [19, 29, 33–35]. In a British multicenter study encompassing 21 centers and 1283 cancer staging reports, Patel et al. showed that compared to 48.7% of narrative reports, 87.3% of SRs contained all required staging information, yielding a 78% improvement in staging completeness at all centers and for all cancer types [35] (Fig. 5.3). Template-based SR has also been shown to be more effective than unstructured reporting for determining tumor resectability, such as in the case of pancreatic adenocarcinoma [36] or rectal cancer [37].

- *Error reduction.* Template-based SR can help reduce the rate of diagnostic errors owing to its ordered structure, allowing radiologists to focus their attention on relevant findings and systematically review the report at the end of the reporting process [19, 24]. In a retrospective analysis of 3000 spine MRI examinations, SR would have revealed 68.6% of extraspinal collateral findings compared to 7.2% actually highlighted by narrative reporting [38]. In a review of 644 radiological reports, Hawkins et al. showed that, compared to narrative reporting, SR enabled a statistically significant reduction of nongrammatical errors (26% vs. 33%, $p = 0.024$), omission errors (i.e., capable of modifying the meaning of a sentence: 1.2% vs. 3.5%, $p = 0.0175$), and commission errors (i.e., due to typos contradicting the report findings or conclusions: 0.8% vs. 3.9%, $p = 0.0007$) [39]. Furthermore, compared to narrative reporting, SR was associated with a greater recall rate of patients with critical findings (i.e., requiring diagnostic or therapeutic intervention: 82.7% vs. 65.1%, $p < 0.001$), implying that the greater communicative efficacy of template-based SR can also have a positive effect in preventing clinical management errors [40].

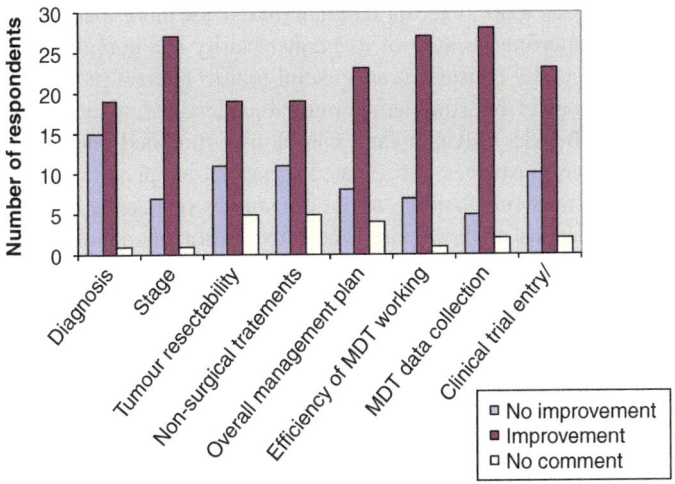

Fig. 5.3 Perceived performance improvement of template-based radiological SR compared to narrative reporting for the diagnostic workup of cancer patients by oncology multidisciplinary team (MDT) end-users, as assessed by Patel et al. [35]. Adapted from [37] under a Creative Commons Attribution Noncommercial license (CC BY-NC 4.0, https://creativecommons.org/licenses/by-nc/4.0/)

5.3 Potential Limitations of Template-Based SR

It has been observed that the adoption of template-based SR can be hampered by several factors, including the following:

- *Resistance to change.* Some radiologists believe that template-based SR is too rigid and may therefore limit their freedom of expression. According to this opinion, template-based SR could involve the risk of worse communication (due to the inability to express useful details for an accurate diagnosis) and reduced consideration of the radiologist's profession compared to other specialists, as it would be seen by nonradiologists as more of a laboratory report than a clinical consultation between colleagues [4, 10, 19, 41]. As a matter of fact, nonradiologists tend to accept template-based SR more than narrative reporting because of its greater clarity and completeness and actually consider it as a useful tool to interact more with radiologists by stimulating mutual understanding and trust [42]. Besides, SR templates can be user-modified under specific circumstances. A dedicated section of template-based SR that leaves full freedom to the operator is represented by the conclusions of the report, where the radiologist summarizes the results of his diagnostic reasoning and offers an interpretation based on the scientific and professional skills pertaining to his/her specialty [10].

- The radiologists' *learning curve* during the transition from narrative reporting to template-based SR might lead to longer turnaround times that could negatively impact workflow and overall productivity. A gradual transition from narrative reporting to SR should be preferred over an abrupt one, prioritizing simpler templates and/or some already validated by scientific societies and institutions. In addition, the learning curve issue would not be due to any intrinsic limitation of template-based SR itself, but rather to a problem of adaptation to change involving individual radiologists to different degrees (i.e., some radiologists would be slower and others faster than average, resulting in a partial compensation effect) [19, 41].

- *Reduced concentration on images* due to the radiologist keeping his/her eyes more focused on the SR template than on images. This argument is supported by psycho-perceptive considerations on the basis that we as humans are accustomed from birth to elaborating visual stimuli and communicating using verbal language. Hence, distracting the radiologist from images could compromise the mental process leading from image observation to diagnosis, involving a higher likelihood of errors, longer reporting times, and reduced productivity [19, 41, 43].

- *Oversimplification*, which might make template-based SR less suitable than narrative reporting for communicating more subtle details or complex information, especially in atypical and/ or more difficult cases [4, 19, 44, 45]. However, SR templates usually include free text fields to cater to any additional data that cannot be embedded in default template fields. The user can also create new templates or adopt more advanced technological solutions allowing for greater template flexibility while maintaining the SR architecture.

- Additional limitations of template-based SR may be related to the presence of unnecessary details (such as in negative templates or simpler cases, compromising the fluency and understability of the report), improper use (possibly causing more errors, e.g., retaining the predefined sentence "no gallbladder stones" in post-cholecystectomy patients), and failure to report collateral findings, as radiologists may focus exclusively on the key features of the disease condition(s) related to the template of their choice, paying scarce attention to unexpected findings [10, 19]. Narrative reporting is not immune to those same issues, which depend on poorer radiologist's attention due, e.g., to tiredness or lack of time. Yet, the hierarchical architecture of template-based SR (including incidental findings and conclusions) should offer an additional safety margin over narrative reporting, in that the various template items can systematically be checked at the end of reporting, thus minimizing the risk of inaccuracies or missing findings.

5.4 Clues for the Implementation of Template-Based Radiological SR

A prerequisite for a successful adoption of template-based SR in radiology is that radiologists do not see it as a potential danger to their professional reputation, but leverage its strengths to improve the quality of their work and prioritize it over mere quantity, lead the transition from narrative reporting to SR, and increase the consideration of their professional role among nonradiologists and patients [46]. A positive attitude toward SR should spur the creation of templates based on validated recommendations and multispecialty involvement of radiologists and nonradiologists [9]. Template-based SRs can also be produced based on existing clinical decision support systems (CDS) that apply validated diagnostic and/or therapeutic pathways to provide recommendations for the diagnosis and subsequent patient management, starting from clinical data and imaging findings [3, 19, 24].

The adoption of template-based SR should begin with a pilot experimentation among most enthusiastic radiologists as a first step to gain familiarity with it and gradually spread the process to the entire workplace. Simpler, more flexible and easily standardizable templates should be preferred in this start-up phase over more complex ones [9, 47], and subspecialty radiological and clinical societies should disseminate up-to-date SR templates for free usage by the medical community [9, 11] (Fig. 5.4). At every facility, SR performance should be regularly audited by radiologists and other specialists to test its effectiveness and fix any potential issues.

The availability of state-of-the-art technology is essential to integrate template-based SR into existing RIS/PACS systems, supporting seamless connection with the identification codes of templates, voice recognition devices, and direct data transfer from DICOM images into the report [4, 23]. Further requirements to fully tap the potential of template-based SR include the option to add links to key images, measurements, and advanced processing data directly into the report (e.g., findings of CAD systems or quantitative biomarkers) [9, 19], and the interoperability with other IT systems (including those handling dematerialized clinical request and informed consent, electronic medical record, radiation dose and contrast medium monitoring, etc.), possibly harnessing the power of cutting-edge artificial intelligence algorithms [48].

Structured MRI report template
primary staging

Local tumour status

- Morphology
  - □ Solid - polypoid
  - □ Solid - (semi-)annular
  - □ Mucinous

- Distance from the anorectal junction to the lower pole of the tumour: .... cm

- Tumour length: .... cm

- T-stage
  - □ T1-2
  - □ T3 → □ T3a or T3b (5 mm extramural growth)
  - □ T3c or T3d (>5 mm extramural growth)
  - □ T4, based on growth into ....

- Sphincter invasion: □ No
  - □ Internal sphincter only
  - □ + intersphincteric plane } □ upper □ middle □ distal 1/3 of anal canal
  - □ + external sphincter

Mesorectal fascia (and peritoneal) involvement

- Shortest distance between tumour and MRF: .... mm → □ free (> 2 mm)
  □ threatened/involved (2 mm)
- Location of the shortest distance between tumour and MRF: .... o'clock
- Relation to anterior peritoneal reflection: □ below (MRF invasion) □ above

Lymph nodes and tumour deposits

- N-stage □ N0 □ N+
- Total number of lymph nodes: ....
- Number of suspicious lymph nodes: .... (......... mesorectal nodes, ... extramesorectal nodes)
  - □ nodes with short axis diameter 9 mm
  - □ nodes with short axis diameter 5–8 mm AND at least 2 morphologic criteria*
  - □ nodes with short axis diameter < 5 mm AND all 3 morphologic criteria*
  *N.B. Morphologic suspicious criteria: [1] round shape, [2] irregular border, [3] heterogenous signal
- Are there any remaining tumour deposits within the mesorectum: □ no, □ yes .... (number of deposits)

Extramural vascular invasion
□ Yes □ No

Structured MRI report template
restaging after neoadjuvant treatment

Local tumour status

- Residual tumour mass:
  - □ No, completely normalised rectal wall (complete response)
  - □ No, fibrotic wall thickening without clear residual mass (complete or near complete response)
  - □ Yes, residual mass (and/or focal high signal on DWI):
    yT-stage □ yT1-2
    □ yT3 → □ yT3a or yT3b (5 mm extramural growth)
    □ yT3c or yT3d (>5 mm extramural growth)
    □ yT4, based on growth into: .... cm

- Distance from the anorectal junction to the lower pole of the tumour .... cm
- Tumour length: .... cm
- Sphincter invasion: □ No
  - □ Internal sphincter only
  - □ + intersphincteric plane } □ upper □ middle □ distal 1/3 of anal canal
  - □ + external sphincter

Mesorectal fascia (and peritoneal) involvement

- Shortest distance between tumour and MRF: .... mm → □ free (> 2 mm)
  □ threatened/involved (2 mm)
- Location of the shortest distance between tumour and MRF: .... o'clock
- Relation to anterior peritoneal reflection: □ below (MRF invasion) □ above

Lymph nodes and tumour deposits

- Lymph nodes □ yN0 = no remaining nodes or only nodes < 5 mm
  □ yN+ = presence of any nodes with a short axis diameter ≥ 5 mm
- Number of residual suspicious (≥ 5 mm) mesorectal lymph nodes: ....
- Number of residual suspicious (≥ 5 mm) extramesorectal lymph nodes: ....
- Are there any remaining tumour deposits within the mesorectum: □ no □ yes .... (number of deposits)

Extramural vascular invasion
□ Yes □ No

Fig. 5.4 SR templates for MRI-based primary staging (left) and post-neoadjuvant treatment restaging of rectal cancer (right) devised by the 2016 ESGAR consensus meeting. Reproduced from [15] under a Creative Commons Attribution 4.0 International license (CC BY 4.0, http://creativecommons.org/licenses/by/4.0/)

References

1. Società Italiana di Radiologia Medica e Interventistica. Atto medico radiologico. https://www.sirm.org/download/184 (in Italian).
2. Larson DB, Froehle CM, Johnson ND, Towbin AJ. Communication in diagnostic radiology: meeting the challenges of complexity. AJR Am J Roentgenol. 2014;203:957–64. https://doi.org/10.2214/AJR.14.12949.
3. Thrall JH. Appropriateness and imaging utilization: "computerized provider order entry and decision support". Acad Radiol. 2014;21:1083–7. https://doi.org/10.1016/j.acra.2014.02.019.
4. Faggioni L, Coppola F, Ferrari R, Neri E, Regge D. Usage of structured reporting in radiological practice: results from an Italian online survey. Eur Radiol. 2017;27:1934–43. https://doi.org/10.1007/s00330-016-4553-6.
5. Nobel JM, Kok EM, Robben SGF. Redefining the structure of structured reporting in radiology. Insights Imaging. 2020;11:10. https://doi.org/10.1186/s13244-019-0831-6.
6. Clunie DA. DICOM structured reporting. Bangor, PA: PixelMed Publishing; 2000. https://www.dclunie.com/pixelmed/DICOMSR.book.zip.
7. Bosmans JM, Neri E, Ratib O, Kahn CE Jr. Structured reporting: a fusion reactor hungry for fuel. Insights Imaging. 2015;6:129–32. https://doi.org/10.1007/s13244-014-0368-7.
8. Noumeir R. Benefits of the DICOM structured report. J Digit Imaging. 2006;19:295–306. https://doi.org/10.1007/s10278-006-0631-7.
9. European Society of Radiology (ESR). ESR paper on structured reporting in radiology. Insights Imaging. 2018;9:1–7. https://doi.org/10.1007/s13244-017-0588-8.
10. Brady AP. Radiology reporting-from Hemingway to HAL? Insights Imaging. 2018;9:237–46. https://doi.org/10.1007/s13244-018-0596-3.
11. Kahn CE Jr, Langlotz CP, Burnside ES, et al. Toward best practices in radiology reporting. Radiology. 2009;252:852–6. https://doi.org/10.1148/radiol.2523081992.
12. Sobez LM, Kim SH, Angstwurm M, et al. Creating high-quality radiology reports in foreign languages through multilingual structured reporting. Eur Radiol. 2019;29:6038–48. https://doi.org/10.1007/s00330-019-06206-8.
13. Beets-Tan RGH, Lambregts DMJ, Maas M, et al. Magnetic resonance imaging for clinical management of rectal cancer: updated recommendations from the 2016 European Society of Gastrointestinal and Abdominal Radiology (ESGAR) consensus meeting. Eur Radiol. 2018;28:1465–75. https://doi.org/10.1007/s00330-017-5026-2.
14. Radiological Society of North America. RadLex®. http://radlex.org/.
15. Clunie DA. DICOM structured reporting and cancer clinical trials results. Cancer Inform. 2007;4:33–56. https://doi.org/10.4137/cin.s37032.

16. Larson DB, Towbin AJ, Pryor RM, Donnelly LF. Improving consistency in radiology reporting through the use of department-wide standardized structured reporting. Radiology. 2013;267:240–50. https://doi.org/10.1148/radiol.12121502.

17. Schwartz LH, Panicek DM, Berk AR, Li Y, Hricak H. Improving communication of diagnostic radiology findings through structured reporting. Radiology. 2011;260:174–81. https://doi.org/10.1148/radiol.11101913.

18. Marcovici PA, Taylor GA. Journal Club: structured radiology reports are more complete and more effective than unstructured reports. AJR Am J Roentgenol. 2014;203:1265–71. https://doi.org/10.2214/AJR.14.12636.

19. Ganeshan D, Duong PT, Probyn L, et al. Structured reporting in radiology. Acad Radiol. 2018;25:66–73. https://doi.org/10.1016/j.acra.2017.08.005.

20. Shea LAG, Towbin AJ. The state of structured reporting: the nuance of standardized language. Pediatr Radiol. 2019;49:500–8. https://doi.org/10.1007/s00247-019-04345-0.

21. Wetterauer C, Winkel DJ, Federer-Gsponer JR, et al. Novices in MRI-targeted prostate biopsy benefit from structured reporting of MRI findings. World J Urol. 2019;38(7):1729–34. https://doi.org/10.1007/s00345-019-02953-x.

22. Ernst BP, Strieth S, Katzer F, et al. The use of structured reporting of head and neck ultrasound ensures time-efficiency and report quality during residency. Eur Arch Otorhinolaryngol. 2020;277:269–76. https://doi.org/10.1007/s00405-019-05679-z.

23. Pinto Dos Santos D, Baeßler B. Big data, artificial intelligence, and structured reporting. Eur Radiol Exp. 2018;2:42. https://doi.org/10.1186/s41747-018-0071-4.

24. Goldberg-Stein S, Chernyak V. Adding value in radiology reporting. J Am Coll Radiol. 2019;16:1292–8. https://doi.org/10.1016/j.jacr.2019.05.042.

25. American College of Radiology. Reporting and data systems. https://www.acr.org/Clinical-Resources/Reporting-and-Data-Systems.

26. Sabel BO, Plum JL, Kneidinger N, et al. Structured reporting of CT examinations in acute pulmonary embolism. J Cardiovasc Comput Tomogr. 2017;11:188–95. https://doi.org/10.1016/j.jcct.2017.02.008.

27. Sabel BO, Plum JL, Czihal M, et al. Structured reporting of CT angiography runoff examinations of the lower extremities. Eur J Vasc Endovasc Surg. 2018;55:679–87. https://doi.org/10.1016/j.ejvs.2018.01.026.

28. Schoeppe F, Sommer WH, Nörenberg D, et al. Structured reporting adds clinical value in primary CT staging of diffuse large B-cell lymphoma. Eur Radiol. 2018;28:3702–9. https://doi.org/10.1007/s00330-018-5340-3.

29. Travis AR, Sevenster M, Ganesh R, Peters JF, Chang PJ. Preferences for structured reporting of measurement data: an institutional survey of medical oncologists, oncology registrars, and radiologists. Acad Radiol. 2014;21:785–96. https://doi.org/10.1016/j.acra.2014.02.008.

30. Bink A, Benner J, Reinhardt J, et al. Structured reporting in neuroradiology: intracranial tumors. Front Neurol. 2018;9:32. https://doi.org/10.3389/fneur.2018.00032.

31. Franconeri A, Fang J, Carney B, et al. Structured vs narrative reporting of pelvic MRI for fibroids: clarity and impact on treatment planning. Eur Radiol. 2018;28:3009–17. https://doi.org/10.1007/s00330-017-5161-9.

32. Ghoshhajra BB, Lee AM, Ferencik M, et al. Interpreting the interpretations: the use of structured reporting improves referring clinicians' comprehension of coronary CT angiography reports. J Am Coll Radiol. 2013;10:432–8. https://doi.org/10.1016/j.jacr.2012.11.012.

33. Nishino M, Jagannathan JP, Ramaiya NH, Van den Abbeele AD. Revised RECIST guideline version 1.1: what oncologists want to know and what radiologists need to know. AJR Am J Roentgenol. 2010;195:281–9. https://doi.org/10.2214/AJR.09.4110.

34. Alkasab TK, Bizzo BC, Berland LL, Nair S, Pandharipande PV, Harvey HB. Creation of an open framework for point-of-care computer-assisted reporting and decision support tools for radiologists. J Am Coll Radiol. 2017;14:1184–9. https://doi.org/10.1016/j.jacr.2017.04.031.

35. Patel A, Rockall A, Guthrie A, et al. Can the completeness of radiological cancer staging reports be improved using proforma reporting? A prospective multicentre non-blinded interventional study across 21 centres in the UK. BMJ Open. 2018;8:e018499. https://doi.org/10.1136/bmjopen-2017-018499.

36. Brook OR, Brook A, Vollmer CM, Kent TS, Sanchez N, Pedrosa I. Structured reporting of multiphasic CT for pancreatic cancer: potential effect on staging and surgical planning. Radiology. 2015;274:464–72. https://doi.org/10.1148/radiol.14140206.

37. Brown PJ, Rossington H, Taylor J, et al. Standardised reports with a template format are superior to free text reports: the case for rectal cancer reporting in clinical practice. Eur Radiol. 2019;29:5121–8. https://doi.org/10.1007/s00330-019-06028-8.

38. Quattrocchi CC, Giona A, Di Martino AC, et al. Extra-spinal incidental findings at lumbar spine MRI in the general population: a large cohort study. Insights Imaging. 2013;4:301–8. https://doi.org/10.1007/s13244-013-0234-z.

39. Hawkins CM, Hall S, Zhang B, Towbin AJ. Creation and implementation of department-wide structured reports: an analysis of the impact on error rate in radiology reports. J Digit Imaging. 2014;27:581–7. https://doi.org/10.1007/s10278-014-9699-7.

40. Buckley BW, Daly L, Allen GN, Ridge CA. Recall of structured radiology reports is significantly superior to that of unstructured reports. Br J Radiol. 2018;91:20170670. https://doi.org/10.1259/bjr.20170670.

41. Weiss DL, Langlotz CP. Structured reporting: patient care enhancement or productivity nightmare? Radiology. 2008;249:739–47. https://doi.org/10.1148/radiol.2493080988.

42. Fatahi N, Krupic F, Hellström M. Difficulties and possibilities in communication between referring clinicians and radiologists: perspective of clinicians. J Multidiscip Healthc. 2019;12:555–64. https://doi.org/10.2147/JMDH.S207649.
43. Srinivasa Babu A, Brooks ML. The malpractice liability of radiology reports: minimizing the risk. Radiographics. 2015;35:547–54. https://doi.org/10.1148/rg.352140046.
44. Baron RL. The radiologist as interpreter and translator. Radiology. 2014;272:4–8. https://doi.org/10.1148/radiol.14140613.
45. Vaché T, Bratan F, Mège-Lechevallier F, Roche S, Rabilloud M, Rouvière O. Characterization of prostate lesions as benign or malignant at multiparametric MR imaging: comparison of three scoring systems in patients treated with radical prostatectomy. Radiology. 2014;272:446–55. https://doi.org/10.1148/radiol.14131584.
46. Bosmans JM, Peremans L, Menni M, De Schepper AM, Duyck PO, Parizel PM. Structured reporting: if, why, when, how-and at what expense? Results of a focus group meeting of radiology professionals from eight countries. Insights Imaging. 2012;3:295–302. https://doi.org/10.1007/s13244-012-0148-1.
47. Larson DB. Strategies for implementing a standardized structured radiology reporting program. Radiographics. 2018;38:1705–16. https://doi.org/10.1148/rg.2018180040.
48. European Society of Radiology (ESR). What the radiologist should know about artificial intelligence—an ESR white paper. Insights Imaging. 2019;10:44. https://doi.org/10.1186/s13244-019-0738-2.

Common Data Elements and Modular Reporting

6

Marc Kohli, Adam Flanders,
Tarik Alkasab, Judy Gichoya,
Ashley Prosper, and Mansoor Fatehi

Contents

M. Kohli (✉)
Department of Radiology and Biomedical Imaging, UCSF,
San Francisco, CA, USA
e-mail: marc.kohli@ucsf.edu

A. Flanders
Department of Radiology, Thomas Jefferson University,
Philadelphia, PA, USA
e-mail: adam.flanders@jefferson.edu

© European Society of Medical Imaging Informatics
(EuSoMII) 2022
M. Fatehi, D. Pinto dos Santos (eds.), *Structured Reporting in Radiology*, Imaging Informatics for Healthcare Professionals,
https://doi.org/10.1007/978-3-030-91349-6_6

119

T. Alkasab
Department of Radiology, Massachusetts General Hospital, Harvard
Medical School, Boston, MA, USA
e-mail: talkasab@mgh.harvard.edu

J. Gichoya
Department of Radiology, Emory University, Atlanta, GA, USA
e-mail: judywawira@emory.edu

A. Prosper
Radiology, UCLA, Los Angeles, CA, USA
e-mail: aprosper@mednet.ucla.edu

M. Fatehi
Biobank, National Brain Mapping Laboratory, Tehran, Iran

6.1   Common Data Elements

6.1.1   Concept

A common data element (CDE) is an attribute of a clinical entity
with a defined semantic label and a defined range of allowed values. The defined semantics and range of allowed values permit a
reliable exchange of information between clinical and research
information systems. Put another way, a CDE is a well-defined
question that might be asked in a specific clinical situation and its
allowed answers. CDEs can be used as labels for data associated
with imaging findings such as specific anatomic location, category of shape, image number, image coordinates, and finding
dimensions. More complex computed values such as texture metrics, areas, volumes, and regions of interest could also be encoded
using CDEs as labels. These standardized, defined, and registered
data element definitions allow radiologists to create structured
descriptions of imaging findings that can be used by downstream
information systems. The CDE project was born out of a joint
meeting of the RSNA and ACR Informatics leaders, where communication of semantically valid findings was identified as a
major informatics gap.

6.1.2 Example

The success of the CDE effort requires the inclusion of concepts, observations, and findings that are relevant to specific clinical use cases, as well as instances in which the inclusion of one or more CDEs improve the fidelity, consistency, and accuracy of the information being conveyed in the clinical report. As such, the creation of CDE content by domain experts is critical to the utility of the effort. Because organized radiology is already represented by subspecialty societies with expertise in specific imaging knowledge and cooperative liaisons with their respective clinical subspecialists, build-out of content should be led by radiology subspecialty organizations in consultation with clinical counterparts. Moreover, subspecialty societies have the experience and knowledge to identify clinical use-cases of high value and utility. These would include imaging concepts/observations that have been proven to have value in the care cycle for grading the severity of disease, predicting treatment response/prognosis, and guiding therapy. Moreover, domain experts are more familiar with existing grading systems that have proven to have reliability in subjective testing. In that regard, the initial outreach for subspecialty expertise began with the American Society of Neuroradiology (ASNR). The ASNR was an early collaborator on related efforts (RadLex and RadReport) and was eager to provide guidance for the assembly of the neuroradiology CDE collection. A team of ASNR volunteers were recruited to participate that have further subspecialty expertise in head and neck, brain, and spine imaging, and each represents a subspecialty organization in neuroradiology (e.g., ASHNR, ASSR, etc.). Initial group meetings were focused upon identifying specific areas of interest, impact, and value and assigning individuals to the creation of draft modules or sets of CDEs that addressed specific clinical use cases. The group reviewed the draft elements and made suggestions and recommendations, and an initial set was posted on the ASNR website for public comment—https://www.asnr.org/resources/cde/ [1]. This initial set consists of 20 modules or sets with roughly 242 individual CDEs. These are in the process of being adapted and published on the

RSNA RadElement site The goal is to repeat this process with other radiology subspecialty organizations and develop a common method for drafting, vetting, curating, and publishing CDEs to the RadElement repository. Readers interested in learning more about the ASNR approach may find [2] a useful resource.

6.1.3 CDE Creation and Lifecycle

The creation and approval process for CDEs and CDE sets was designed to parallel the peer-review process for journal articles. Additionally, we have built on lessons learned from the RSNA report template collection. Prospective authors are directed to review the authoring guide posted on https://radelement.org prior to beginning the authoring process.

CDE authors submit new sets and elements to radelement.org either through the API or by using an authoring tool such as ACR MARVAL (Fig. 6.1) { | anon. ACR Assist | MARVAL, no date | | |zu:25445:JXWV7PZ7}.

Sets and elements submitted are immediately assigned a unique identifier (RDESXXXX for sets and RDEXXXX for elements) and are placed into the proposed status. Proposed sets and elements are reviewed by the CDE steering committee, and feedback is provided to the original authors. Feedback is based on the radelement build guidelines, which are also available on radelement.org. These build guidelines are more specific than the author guidelines and cover a number of important topics to drive CDE quality and enable reuse. As a part of the review process, proposed CDEs may be deleted. If a set or data element is deleted from the proposed status, its ID remains reserved but the definition is removed from the repository.

After revisions, the CDE committee approves sets and elements, which then become published. Once published, elements can only be retired and not deleted or modified in order to maintain historical validity.

The CDE project, schema, and radelement.org API are open to using a number of products and services following steering committee approval. One such service is the ACR MARVAL authoring

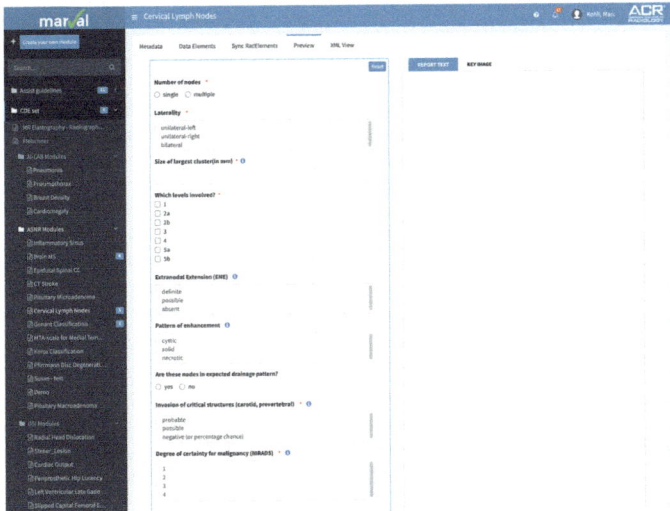

Fig. 6.1 Screenshot from ACR MARVAL application demonstrating the authoring and reviewing view for the Cervical Lymph Nodes CDE set

tool, which has been jointly developed by the CDE steering committee (Fig. 6.1).

MARVAL is a web application that allows the authoring of CDEs, as well as support of the review process. MARVAL walks authors through a stepwise process of creating a new set, providing the required metadata, and then defining individual elements. New elements can be designed from scratch or imported from existing sets. Users are presented with suggestions of existing elements when creating new elements to encourage reuse.

Throughout the process, MARVAL allows for granular comparison of local content with the radelement repository, and after approval, it allows synchronization with a few clicks (Fig. 6.2).

6.1.4   CDE Schema

CDEs can be represented in either extensible markup language (XML) or javascript object notation (JSON) formats, with JSON

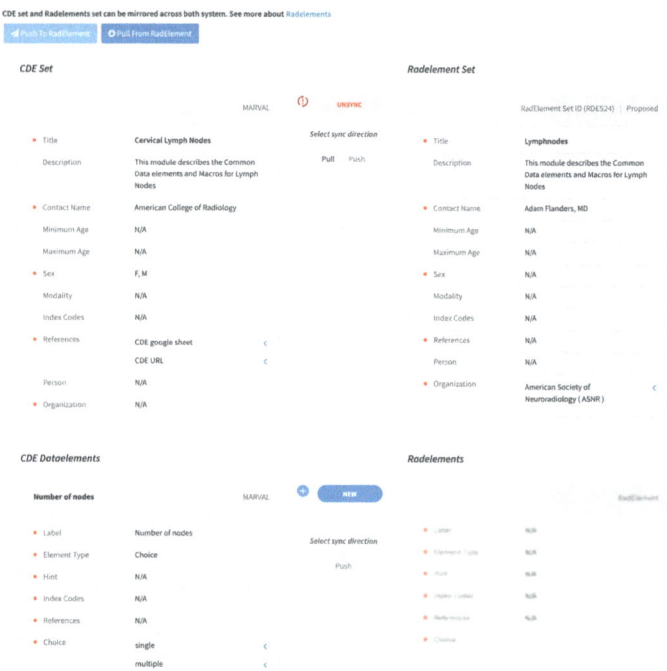

Fig. 6.2 Screenshot from ACR MARVAL application demonstrating synchronization of local changes (left) with radelement.org (right)

preferred. The CDE schema [3] defines how the XML and JSON representations of a CDE are formatted in order to be valid.

The schema is written in the Relax NG compact syntax [4] and builds on the early experience using a data definition language to define the structure and content for radiology report templates [5]. The schema is a starting point for developers who are interested in working with the CDEs programmatically as well as the ACR and RSNA developers who are building canonical CDE tools.

The schema definition starts with defining the top-level of our organizational tree: data_element_set.

```
element data_element_set {
    element id { xsd:string { pattern='RDES\d+' } },
        element name { text },
        element description { text >>
    a:documentation ["plain text, or XHTML div are
    acceptable"]},
        version,
        references?,
        index_codes?,
        element images { image+ }?,
        modality*,
        biological_sex?,
        age_range?,
        authors?,
        history+,
        specialty+,
        element elements { data_element+ }
}
```

The schema requires valid CDE sets to include an id, name, description, and version and a number of optional elements (e.g., references, index_codes). Version, references, and index_codes are examples of named patterns that are defined near the bottom of the schema; the version definition is listed below.

```
version =
        element version {
            element name {text},
            status_attrs
    }


status_attrs =
        element date { xsd:date },
        element status {
          "proposed" | "published" | "retired"
    }
```

Version references another named pattern, status_attrs, which includes a date stamp and the three statuses that are valid for CDE sets, and CDEs are described in the section on authoring.

The modality, biological_sex, and age_range metadata elements are searchable fields that allow a client discovering CDE sets to limit results based on the context of a specific use case.

The authors element allows for 0...n person and organization elements.

```
authors =
        element authors {
            person*, org*
        }

person =
      element person {
        element name { text },
        (element orcid_id { text }?
         & element twitter_handle { text }*
         & element url { text }*
         & element role
    *)
      }
    org =
      element organization {
        element name { text }
        & element abbreviation { text }?
        & element url { xsd:anyURI }?
        & element comment { text }?
        & element role
    *
  }
```

Person and org are structured to provide flexibility tracking both individual and organizational contributions to both CDE sets and CDEs.

Index codes are used to link CDEs to RadLex, Snomed-CT, and Loinc.

```
index_codes =
      element index_codes {
        element index_code {
          element system { "RADLEX" | "SNOMEDCT" |
    "LOINC" },
          element code { xsd:normalizedString },
          element url { xsd:anyURI }?,
          element display { text }?
        }+
    }
```

The index codes array holds 0...n index_code elements, which specify a coding system, the specific code, and URL for the coding system and code and display text for human readability.

Finally, the data element set has an array that holds 1...n CDEs. The schema definition for a CDE is below.

```
data_element =


  element element {
        element id { xsd:string { pattern='RDE\d+'
    } },
        element parent_set { xsd:string {
    pattern='RDES\d+' } },
        element name { text },
        element definition { text },
        version,
        references?,
        index_codes?,
        element images { image+ }?,
        modality*,
        biological_sex?,
        age_range?,
        authors?,
        history+,
        specialty*,
        (
```

```
            element integer_values {
                element min { xsd:integer }?,
                element max { xsd:integer }?,
                element step { xsd:integer >>
    a:documentation ["Default is 1"] }?,
                element unit { xsd:Name }?
            }
            | element float_values {
                element min { xsd:float }?,
                element max { xsd:float }?,
                element step { xsd:integer }?,
                element unit { xsd:Name }?
            }
            | element boolean_values { xsd:boolean
    }
            | element value_set {
                element min_cardinality {
    xsd:nonNegativeInteger }?,
                element max_cardinality {
    xsd:positiveInteger }?,
                element value {
                    element value { xsd:Name },
                    element name { text },
                    element definition { text }?,
                    references?,
                    element images { image+ }?,
                    index_codes?
                }+
            }
        )
    }
```

Many of the metadata elements that define the CDE set are intentionally repeated in the CDE definition. While this may seem redundant, it has been found valuable to model the complexity of imaging.

The most important point to take away from the CDE definition is that there are four types: integer, float, boolean, and value set. Integer and float both have metadata to support basic validation.

The value set is one of the most commonly used CDE types and can be used for both single and multi-select data types by setting min and max cardinality. A single-select (radio button) value set would have a max_cardinality of 1 and, if it is a required field, a min_cardinality of 1. A multi-select (checkbox) would have a max_cardinality of >1 and a min_cardinality of >1 if required.

Value sets are made of individual values that have unique values, names, and definitions and include optional references, exemplar images, and index_codes.

As we built the authoring process, we identified that the reuse of CDEs in new sets required a specification for where the CDE is editable and where it is simply reused. We added the concept of a parent_set, which is the context in which a CDE is editable. With this understanding of the CDE schema, we move on to describing applications.

6.1.5 Applications

6.1.5.1 Artificial Intelligence Integration

Successful AI development is dependent on providing a system with a sufficient volume of accurately annotated and verified data [6]. Data curation is often limited by small sample sizes and the cost- and time-intensive steps required for proper annotation [7]. Ideally, radiology reports generated for clinical care would directly feed AI development. Leveraging existing reports is particularly important in AI development for infrequently encountered pathology and generalizability. Aggregating clinical report data from multiple institutions would address both of these complex problems; however, it is not currently feasible as the vast majority of radiology reports are written in a free-text, narrative style. This unstructured, free-form reporting limits accessibility of data-rich radiology reports for automated analysis. Preparation of free-text reports for use in artificial intelligence (AI) development can be achieved through manual labeling, natural language processing, and deep learning techniques, each with unique pros and cons [8]. Integration of CDEs into the radiology report optimizes the process of AI data curation, facilitating the direct input of clinically derived radiology reports into AI development, training, and validation [6, 9].

6.1.5.2 Decision Support

Electronic decision support tools offer a means of delivering evidence-based follow-up and reporting guidelines to radiologists in real time as they generate reports. When successfully implemented, decision support tools have the potential to promote consistency and reproducibility among radiologists, improve the quality of patient care, improve cost control, and engender trust in referring physicians who receive our reports [10]. Consider the management of incidental pulmonary nodules. More than 1.5 million adult Americans are estimated to have a pulmonary nodule identified each year [11]. Despite being one of the most widely accepted and recognized radiology follow-up guidelines, the Fleischner Society Criteria for pulmonary nodule follow-up [12] are variably utilized with reports of adherence as low as 34% [13]. Structured reporting utilizing CDE to describe incidentally detected nodules proposes structured data fields for describing nodules: size (<6 mm, 6–8 mm, >8 mm), texture (solid, part-solid, ground glass), and multiplicity. In addition to these characteristics of the findings, data elements are provided for patient characteristics: age and smoking history. Together, these provide sufficient information to allow an integrated decision support system to propose guideline-compliant follow-up recommendations (including timing) for these incidental nodules in the imaging report.

In addition to improving follow-up recommendations in the impression section of a radiology report based on its findings section, CDE implementation has the potential to aid radiologists in the way that findings are reported. Inclusion of recommended standardized features and observations deemed necessary for a complete report could be "triggered" by keywords such as "mass" [2, 14]. The American College of Radiology's ACR Assist platform facilitates the inclusion of clinical practice guidelines in radiology reports using rule-based guidelines [14]. Core components included are structured reporting of the "RADS" classification systems (BI-RADS, LungRADS, LI-RADS, PI-RADS) and decision pathways from a myriad of incidental finding white papers [15–25].

6.1.5.3 Trending over Time (Flowsheets)

Many patients receive serial imaging examinations for acute and chronic conditions. Tracking the evolution of a disease process and response to treatment is crucial for the appropriate direction of patient care and informs long-term ability to improve management through retrospective analysis. In the absence of CDE, assessing longitudinal response over serial examinations utilizing heterogeneous reporting styles can be incredibly challenging [26]. Consider oncologic imaging reports where tumor assessment criteria and measurement reporting can vary by institution, cancer type, and research protocol [27]. While surveys of oncologists reveal high expectations for quantitative tumor reporting, radiologists at the same institutions admit the process of incorporating quantitative data into reports to be time-consuming [28, 29]. While most oncologic radiology reports ultimately include information necessary for tracking lesions with Response Evaluation Criteria in Solid Tumors (RECIST) measurements, mining this data can be cumbersome [6]. By utilizing a CDE question/answer structure, tumor measurements can be discreetly stored and transmitted to other systems for analysis.

6.1.5.4 Registry Participation/Submission

The rapid evolution of health information technology with widespread implementation of electronic health records has resulted in the generation of massive amounts of digital patient data and facilitated retrospective and prospective generation of registries with significantly reduced cost [30]. Increased availability of digital data has increased usage of registries in basic research, clinical trials, and the assessment of clinical care quality and efficacy. Comparing institutional performance at the local, regional, and national levels facilitates the identification of areas for process improvement [31]. Quality improvement through registry participation is becoming an increasingly important component for reimbursement. The Center for Medicare and Medicaid Services' National Coverage Decision (NCD) approving lung cancer screening with low-dose CT in 2015 requires imaging facilities to submit data to a CMS-approved registry for each lung cancer screening LDCT that is performed [32]. While lung cancer screening with LDCT is unique in its registry submission requirements being directly linked to reimbursement, CMS has more widely incentivized the use of Qualified Clinical Data Registries (QCDR) through the Medicare Access and CHIP (Children's Health Insurance Program) Reauthorization Act (MACRA) [33]. Participation in CMS-approved QCDRs such as the American College of Radiology's National Radiology Data Registry (NRDR) fulfills requirements for CMS' Merit-Based Incentive Payment System (MIPS). The ACR Lung Cancer Screening Registry (LCSR), National Mammography Database, CT Colonography Registry, and Dose Index Registry are just a few of the registries available for facilitating radiology quality improvement requirements. Regardless of the specific focus of a particular registry, commonly accepted and agreed-upon data elements are its building blocks.

Clearly defining and accurately capturing data elements for inclusion in a registry is critical to its ultimate validity and quality { | anon. Registries for Evaluating Patient Outcomes: A User's Guide: Prior Editions | Effective Health Care Program, no date | | |zu:25445:5NRIYP33}. Consider the ACR LCSR as an example. Patient demographics, medical history, risk factors (including smoking status), LungRads score and information about the scanner used, radiation dose provided, and reading radiologist are just some of the elements that must be provided for each LCS LDCT performed. Because of the highly variable ways in which this data is presented and recorded across institutions, each site is responsible for recording required data elements into the ACR LCSR, often requiring significant manual data mining and input [6]. Alternatively, through the implementation of CDEs directly into radiology reporting templates, data within the radiology report can be easily identified and recorded into a registry [14].

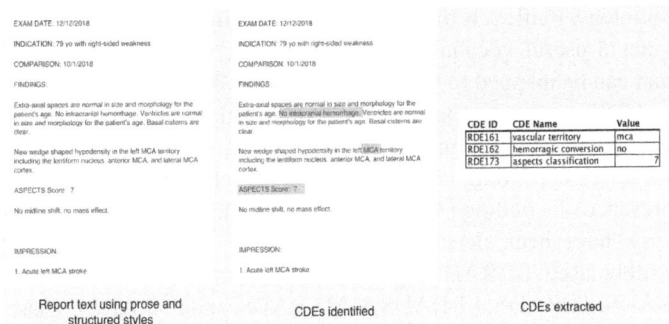

Fig. 6.3 Representation of our desired future-state where radiology reports can contain both free-text elements and structured CDEs

6.2   Modular Reporting

6.2.1   Interaction with RadReport, RadLex, and Other Lexicons

When learning about CDEs, a common question arises regarding how CDEs interact with reporting templates and terminologies such as RadLex or SNOMED-CT.

Reporting templates, such as those stored on RadReport.org, offer the ability to incorporate both free-text elements along with structured questions with finite answer choices through the incorporation of CDEs. The CDE effort is unlikely to cover the entire field of imaging and to keep up with the pace of advances, such that there will always be a place for free text in radiology reports. The combination of report templates and CDEs offers radiologists flexibility in the reporting style of the radiologists by ensuring the most important factors are captured irrespective of whether the report is structured or in free narrative form, as shown in Fig. 6.3.

CDEs can be thought of as pick lists or numeric fill-in fields of dictation systems. They can be invoked during voice dictation to describe a specific finding or set of findings. As CDEs consist of a clinical question with specified allowable answers, the components of each CDE can be mapped to a specific terminology. For radiology, RadLex is the lexicon developed by the RSNA that provides a useful vocabulary for radiologists. Other terminologies that can be mapped to CDEs include SNOMED and LOINC.

CDEs are a core component of contextual structured reporting, whereby different templates are used for various specific clinical scenarios depending on imaging protocol, clinical history, or the presence of a finding [34]. In recent years, more classification systems have been developed for radiology studies, beyond the widely used BI-RADS systems as discussed above (e.g., NI-RADS, TI-RADS, LI-RADS, CAD-RADS, and PI-RADS). These classification systems are usually presented as guidelines, without direction on how to integrate them into the routine reporting workflow. CDEs provide the mechanism for operationalizing such classification systems. For example, the American Society of Neuroradiology (ASNR) has been working closely with the American College of Radiology and RSNA to develop CDEs, with a detailed description of three published CDEs on sinus drainage, neck lymph nodes, and laryngeal cancer [2, 9]. Radelement.org serves as a comprehensive library for imaging CDEs, which are available both in human-readable format and through an API, but at the moment of this writing, most radiology reporting systems have automated easy ingestion of CDEs directly

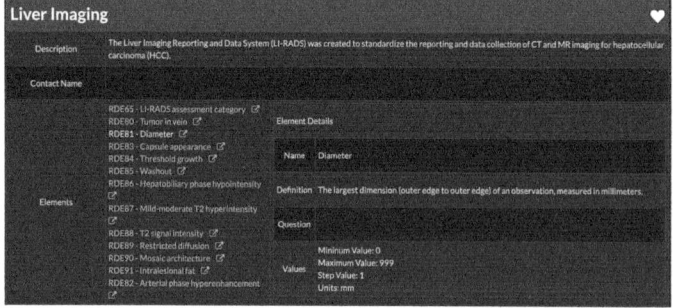

Fig. 6.4 Screenshot from radelement.org depicting the CDE set for LI-RADS, with associated elements. The RDE81—Diameter element is selected and displayed in the right-hand pane of the web page

from radelement.org. Therefore, integration into dictation systems falls to the local informatics team for initial installation and periodic maintenance.

Figure 6.4 shows an example CDE from radelement.org set that captures the elements in the LI-RADS classification of liver lesions [35].

For each element in the CDE, there is a detailed description and definition and expected values including maximum and minimum limits. The design of most CDEs is such that they are modality agnostic, with most elements usable across CT and MRI imaging.

Due to the detailed nature of structured text reporting, which can include multiple CDEs, radiologists can be more prone to error from eye dwell when they focus on the text to be completed rather than the medical images [36]. While the majority of CDEs are a result of radiologist interpretations, the CDE structure can be easily integrated into DICOM SR and FHIR objects, which would allow for an AI model to discreetly present findings to a radiologist to validate before inclusion in the final report. CDEs are envisioned as a key component for the efficient integration of AI into the radiologist workflow. With the semantic knowledge in a CDE, a reporting vendor could link particular phrases or groups of words together with a particular CDE or result from an AI model. For example, by dictating or measuring an adrenal mass or a lymph node, the reporting system could contextually launch the relevant CDE and prepopulate the relevant information into the radiology report saving valuable time and decreasing transcription errors.

6.3   Conclusion

In conclusion, the RSNA/ACR CDEs provide a schema definition, central repository, and editing and curation tools, which enable the collection, storage, and transmission of discrete, clinically actionable, and relevant information from imaging studies.

References

1. CDE. ASNR. https://www.asnr.org/resources/cde/. Accessed 15 Sept 2020.
2. Flanders AE, Jordan JE. The ASNR-ACR-RSNA common data elements project: what will it do for the house of neuroradiology? Am J Neuroradiol. 2019;40:14–8. https://doi.org/10.3174/ajnr.A5780.
3. RadElement.org—Common Data Elements (CDE) for radiology. http://radelement.org/. Accessed 31 Aug 2017.
4. RELAX NG home page. https://relaxng.org/. Accessed 27 July 2020.
5. Bozkurt S, Kahn CE. An open-standards grammar for outline-style radiology report templates. J Digit Imaging. 2012;25:359–64. https://doi.org/10.1007/s10278-012-9456-8.
6. Kohli M, Alkasab T, Wang K, et al. Bending the artificial intelligence curve for radiology: informatics tools from ACR and RSNA. J Am Coll Radiol. 2019;16:1464–70. https://doi.org/10.1016/j.jacr.2019.06.009.
7. Willemink MJ, Koszek WA, Hardell C, et al. Preparing medical imaging data for machine learning. Radiology. 2020;295:4–15. https://doi.org/10.1148/radiol.2020192224.
8. Chen MC, Ball RL, Yang L, et al. Deep learning to classify radiology free-text reports. Radiology. 2017;286:845–52. https://doi.org/10.1148/radiol.2017171115.
9. Rajamohan AG, Patel V, Sheikh-Bahaei N, et al. Common data elements in head and neck radiology reporting. Neuroimaging Clin N Am. 2020;30:379–91. https://doi.org/10.1016/j.nic.2020.05.002.
10. Boland GWL, Thrall JH, Gazelle GS, et al. Decision support for radiologist report recommendations. J Am Coll Radiol. 2011;8:819–23. https://doi.org/10.1016/j.jacr.2011.08.003.
11. Gould MK, Tang T, Liu I-LA, et al. Recent trends in the identification of incidental pulmonary nodules. Am J Respir Crit Care Med. 2015;192:1208–14. https://doi.org/10.1164/rccm.201505-0990OC.
12. MacMahon H, Naidich DP, Goo JM, et al. Guidelines for management of incidental pulmonary nodules detected on CT images: from the Fleischner Society 2017. Radiology. 2017;284:228–43. https://doi.org/10.1148/radiol.2017161659.
13. Lacson R, Prevedello LM, Andriole KP, et al. Factors associated with radiologists' adherence to Fleischner Society guidelines for management of pulmonary nodules. J Am Coll Radiol JACR. 2012;9:468–73. https://doi.org/10.1016/j.jacr.2012.03.009.
14. Rubin DL, Kahn CE. Common data elements in radiology. Radiology. 2016;283:837–44. https://doi.org/10.1148/radiol.2016161553.
15. Munden RF, Carter BW, Chiles C, et al. Managing incidental findings on thoracic CT: mediastinal and cardiovascular findings. A white paper of the ACR Incidental Findings Committee. J Am Coll Radiol JACR. 2018;15:1087–96. https://doi.org/10.1016/j.jacr.2018.04.029.

16. Berland LL, Silverman SG, Gore RM, et al. Managing incidental findings on abdominal CT: white paper of the ACR Incidental Findings Committee. J Am Coll Radiol. 2010;7:754–73. https://doi.org/10.1016/j.jacr.2010.06.013.
17. Patel MD, Ascher SM, Horrow MM, et al. Management of incidental adnexal findings on CT and MRI: a white paper of the ACR Incidental Findings Committee. J Am Coll Radiol JACR. 2020;17:248–54. https://doi.org/10.1016/j.jacr.2019.10.008.
18. Hoang JK, Hoffman AR, González RG, et al. Management of incidental pituitary findings on CT, MRI, and 18F-fluorodeoxyglucose PET: a white paper of the ACR Incidental Findings Committee. J Am Coll Radiol JACR. 2018;15:966–72. https://doi.org/10.1016/j.jacr.2018.03.037.
19. Megibow AJ, Baker ME, Morgan DE, et al. Management of incidental pancreatic cysts: a white paper of the ACR Incidental Findings Committee. J Am Coll Radiol JACR. 2017;14:911–23. https://doi.org/10.1016/j.jacr.2017.03.010.
20. Mayo-Smith WW, Song JH, Boland GL, et al. Management of incidental adrenal masses: a white paper of the ACR Incidental Findings Committee. J Am Coll Radiol. 2017;14:1038–44. https://doi.org/10.1016/j.jacr.2017.05.001.
21. Herts BR, Silverman SG, Hindman NM, et al. Management of the incidental renal mass on CT: a white paper of the ACR Incidental Findings Committee. J Am Coll Radiol. 2018;15:264–73. https://doi.org/10.1016/j.jacr.2017.04.028.
22. Gore RM, Pickhardt PJ, Mortele KJ, et al. Management of incidental liver lesions on CT: a white paper of the ACR Incidental Findings Committee. J Am Coll Radiol. 2017;14:1429–37. https://doi.org/10.1016/j.jacr.2017.07.018.
23. Hoang JK, Langer JE, Middleton WD, et al. Managing incidental thyroid nodules detected on imaging: white paper of the ACR Incidental Thyroid Findings Committee. J Am Coll Radiol. 2015;12:143–50. https://doi.org/10.1016/j.jacr.2014.09.038.
24. Berland LL. Overview of white papers of the ACR Incidental Findings Committee II on adnexal, vascular, splenic, nodal, gallbladder, and biliary findings. J Am Coll Radiol JACR. 2013;10:672–4. https://doi.org/10.1016/j.jacr.2013.05.012.
25. Patel MD, Ascher SM, Paspulati RM, et al. Managing incidental findings on abdominal and pelvic CT and MRI, part 1: white paper of the ACR Incidental Findings Committee II on adnexal findings. J Am Coll Radiol JACR. 2013;10:675–81. https://doi.org/10.1016/j.jacr.2013.05.023.
26. Haacke EM, Duhaime AC, Gean AD, et al. Common data elements in radiologic imaging of traumatic brain injury. J Magn Reson Imaging. 2010;32:516–43. https://doi.org/10.1002/jmri.22259.
27. Folio LR, Nelson CJ, Benjamin M, et al. Quantitative radiology reporting in oncology: survey of oncologists and radiologists. Am J Roentgenol. 2015;205:W233–43. https://doi.org/10.2214/AJR.14.14054.

28. Jaffe TA, Wickersham NW, Sullivan DC. Quantitative imaging in oncology patients: part 1, radiology practice patterns at major U.S. Cancer Centers. Am J Roentgenol. 2010;195:101–6. https://doi.org/10.2214/AJR.09.2850.

29. Jaffe TA, Wickersham NW, Sullivan DC. Quantitative imaging in oncology patients: part 2, oncologists' opinions and expectations at major U.S. Cancer Centers. Am J Roentgenol. 2010;195:W19–30. https://doi.org/10.2214/AJR.09.3541.

30. Miller RS, Mitchell K, Myslinski R, Rising J. Health Information Technology (IT) and patient registries. Agency for Healthcare Research and Quality (US); 2019.

31. Patti JA. The National Radiology Data Registry: a necessary component of quality health care. J Am Coll Radiol. 2011;8:453. https://doi.org/10.1016/j.jacr.2011.05.014.

32. Decision Memo for Screening for Lung Cancer with Low Dose Computed Tomography (LDCT) (CAG-00439N). https://www.cms.gov/medicare-coverage-database/details/nca-decision-memo.aspx?NCAId=274. Accessed 10 Aug 2020.

33. Chen MM, Rosenkrantz AB, Nicola GN, et al. The qualified clinical data registry: a pathway to success within MACRA. Am J Neuroradiol. 2017;38:1292–6. https://doi.org/10.3174/ajnr.A5220.

34. Olthof AW, Leusveld ALM, de Groot JC, et al. Contextual structured reporting in radiology: implementation and long-term evaluation in improving the communication of critical findings. J Med Syst. 2020;44:148. https://doi.org/10.1007/s10916-020-01609-3.

35. RadElement Set—Liver Imaging (RDES5). https://radelement.org/home/sets/set/RDES5. Accessed 10 Aug 2020.

36. Srinivasa Babu A, Brooks ML. The malpractice liability of radiology reports: minimizing the risk. Radiographics. 2015;35:547–54. https://doi.org/10.1148/rg.352140046.

Multimedia-Enhanced Structured Reporting

7

David J. Vining

Contents

D. J. Vining (✉)
Diagnostic Radiology, Department of Abdominal Imaging,
University of Texas MD Anderson Cancer Center, Houston, TX, USA
e-mail: dvining@visionsr.com; dvining@mdanderson.org

© European Society of Medical Imaging Informatics (EuSoMII) 2022
M. Fatehi, D. Pinto dos Santos (eds.), *Structured Reporting in Radiology*, Imaging Informatics for Healthcare Professionals, https://doi.org/10.1007/978-3-030-91349-6_7

Multimedia-enhanced structured reporting (MESR) is an advanced form of communication that combines structured elements (i.e., templates and standardized language) with images, video, charts, tables, graphics, and audio in an interactive environment to improve the communication of information. Various names exist for describing MESR including multimedia structured reporting (MSR), multimedia-enhanced radiology reporting (MERR), multimedia interactive content reporting (MMICR), and interactive multimedia reporting (IMR) [1]. Regardless of the acronym, the concept is that multimedia increases cognition and retention, thus enhancing the ability of healthcare providers and patients to comprehend medical information [2–4].

In 2020, a workgroup was formed by the Healthcare Information and Management Systems Society (HIMSS) and the Society for Imaging Informatics in Medicine (SIIM) that began exploring the state-of-the-art of IMR and outlining the technical challenges hindering its adoption [5]. Although MESR is applicable to many medical specialties, adoption has been slow due to a number of technical, human, and economic factors. The growing use of personal activity trackers and medical monitoring devices with multimedia feedback will influence MESR development, but the transition from traditional fee-for-service to value-based healthcare should drive its adoption [6, 7].

7.1 Historical Development

Initial elements of MESR appeared a few years after Roentgen's discovery of X-rays in 1895 with the introduction of illustrated clinical reports [8]. Synoptic reporting started in the early twentieth century with Ernest A. Codman's "end result idea" for creating disease registries but did not gain acceptance until the end of the century [9, 10]. The first synoptic reporting in radiology, attributed to Harold J. Pierce, was described in 1922 [11]. The concepts of "hypertext" and "hypermedia," essential components of interactive multimedia communication, were introduced by Nelson in 1965 but did materialize until the arrival of desktop computers in the 1980s [12]. Early applications of hypermedia were in educational systems that allowed users to access databases and retrieve information including video, sound, and text, and those principles have carried forward into modern MESR [13, 14].

One of the earliest attempts to transform radiology reports into a machine-readable format was in 1965 with a system called MEDTRAN that used a paper tape coding system [15]. A solution that more closely resembled today's MESR was introduced by Schramm in 1989 that presented an animated radiology report for the communication of radiographic findings between radiology and emergency departments [16, 17]. In 1994, Bellon developed a multimedia reporting system that inserted hyperlinks in dictated radiology reports, which accessed annotated images referenced to findings [18]. Bellon's system was built using a DEC 5000 series UNIX workstation (Digital Equipment Corporation, Maynard, MA) capable of recording speech, but he predicted that the widespread use of multimedia reporting was unlikely until "… there is pervasive introduction of computer technology."

In 2001, Vining created an interactive multimedia structured reporting system, called REX™, which recorded key images of radiographic findings and labeled each with metadata using an ontology (i.e., controlled vocabulary with defined relationships between terms) to describe the anatomical location, observation/diagnosis, and secondary characteristics (i.e., details) of the diagnosis (Fig. 7.1) [19]. The system was built using a proprietary image viewer that allowed a user to click on an image to record the finding in a database along with associated measurements, image annotations, and audio voice descriptions. A user had to employ a series of pull-down menus with hierarchies of terminology to label each finding with the appropriate terminology.

In parallel with diagnostic radiology, other medical disciplines began to develop MESR solutions at the same time. In cardiology, Brower developed a computer-based cardiac catheterization data management system in 1987 that included reporting capabilities with graphical analysis of ventricular function [20]. In 1995, Cheng created a multimedia cardiac angiogram tool, called MCAT, which allowed for the annotation of cardiac angiograms with audio, text, and graphics [21]. In 2002, Balogh described a

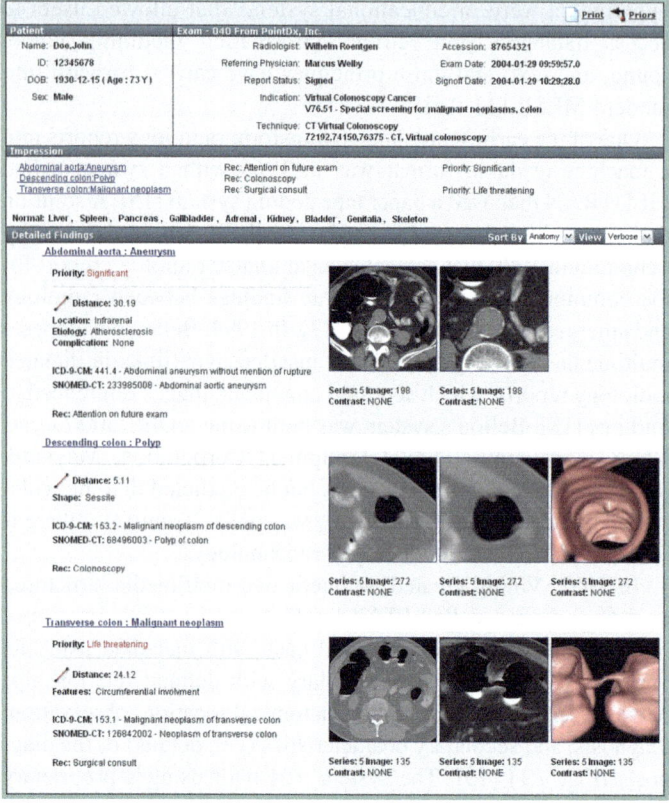

Fig. 7.1 PointDx's multimedia structured report, circa 2004, containing key images tagged with metadata describing the anatomy, pathology, and secondary details

telemedicine architecture, called SAMTA (scalable architecture for medical multimedia telecommunication applications), which delivered cardiac digital image loops and multimedia reports over the Internet using DICOM and MPEG2 video compression [22]. However, these early attempts to build MESR solutions as well as those in other fields were short-lived or limited to academic pursuits due to challenges that persist even today.

7.2   Current State-of-the-Art

Various forms of MESR are continuing to emerge in medical disciplines that use multimedia content to document disease and treatment response, with some of these solutions now becoming commercial products that interface to or integrate with the electronic health record (EHR).

7.2.1   Gastroenterology

Olympus America (Center Valley, PA) offered one of the first commercially available MESR products in the 1990s with its EndoWorks® that documented endoscopic procedures with a combination of free text, synoptic reporting, and endoscopic images; however, the product was discontinued in 2018 [23, 24]. ProVation Medical (Minneapolis, MN) and others have filled the gap with a similar MESR solution (Fig. 7.2) [25]. The adoption of

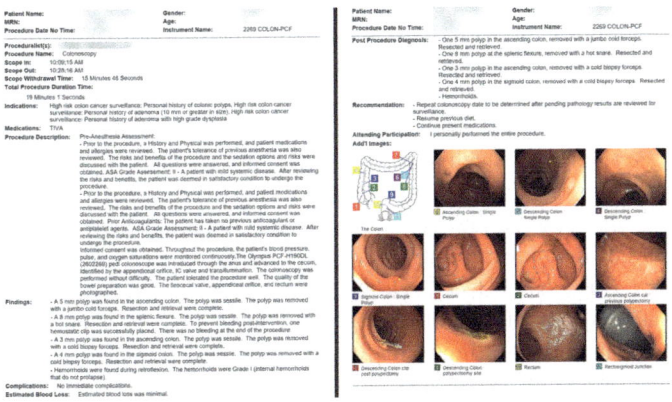

Fig. 7.2 Provation Medical report documenting a colonoscopy procedure with images of multiple polyps found throughout the colon. Additional images document a polyp removal and absence of immediate complications. (Courtesy of Dr. Gottumukkala Raju, MD Anderson Cancer Center, Houston, Texas, USA)

multimedia reporting by gastroenterologists is more widespread than in other imaging fields due to the need to document procedures at the point of care with annotated images and video clips. The limited reporting needs of these dedicated procedures may have facilitated adoption. Unfortunately, endoscopic MESR reports generated by proprietary systems are transmitted to the EHR as a portable document format (PDF) report where the interactive nature of the more advanced MESR solutions is often lost. The technical challenge of transferring the interactivity of MESR solutions to an EHR is one of the tasks that the HIMMS-SIIM IMR workgroup is addressing today.

7.2.2 Cardiology

During the past decade, multiple national and international societies have published policies and guidelines advocating for the adoption of structured reporting in cardiology, but widespread acceptance of even basic, non-MESR structured reporting remains limited [26, 27]. Researchers continue to push the limits with the development of innovative methods for data input into cardiology MESR [28, 29]. Innovation is fostered by the growing awareness that structured reporting will enable big data initiatives that in turn will shape the future of medicine [30].

Commercial imaging vendors began introducing MESR products for use in cardiac catheterization and echocardiography during the past several years to connect multiple elements of cardiovascular care with data from the EHR to improve patient care (Fig. 7.3) [31–33]. Despite these promising advances, the vast majority of cardiology reporting today remains as unstructured narratives of image findings. Furthermore, the challenge of interoperability between proprietary MESR systems and different EHRs remains a barrier confronting cardiology and other image-based medical disciplines.

7.2.3   Radiation Oncology

Radiation oncology relies on image guidance for the delivery of a radiation dose at a particular location and for a specific duration. Treatment planning involves the computation of volumes from cross-sectional images outlining the targeted tissue, dosimetric calculations, and evaluation of dose distribution that is often documented using MESR. The first dose-planning system was devel-

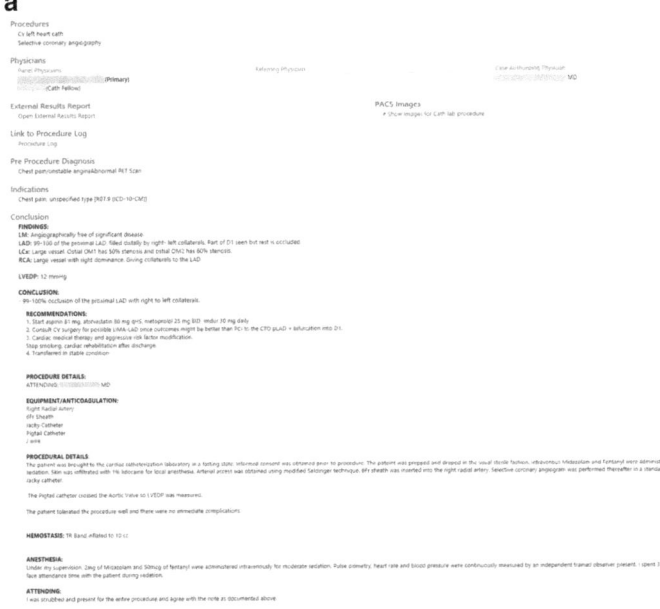

Fig. 7.3 (**a**) Cardiac catheterization structured report with data arranged in a template and presented in tables and with a graphic illustrating sites of disease. (Courtesy of Dr. Sachin Goel, Houston Methodist Hospital, Houston, Texas, USA). (**b**) Cardiac catheterization report includes a graphic of the coronary artery system with locations and degrees of stenosis. (Courtesy of Dr. Sachin Goel, Houston Methodist Hospital, Houston, Texas, USA)

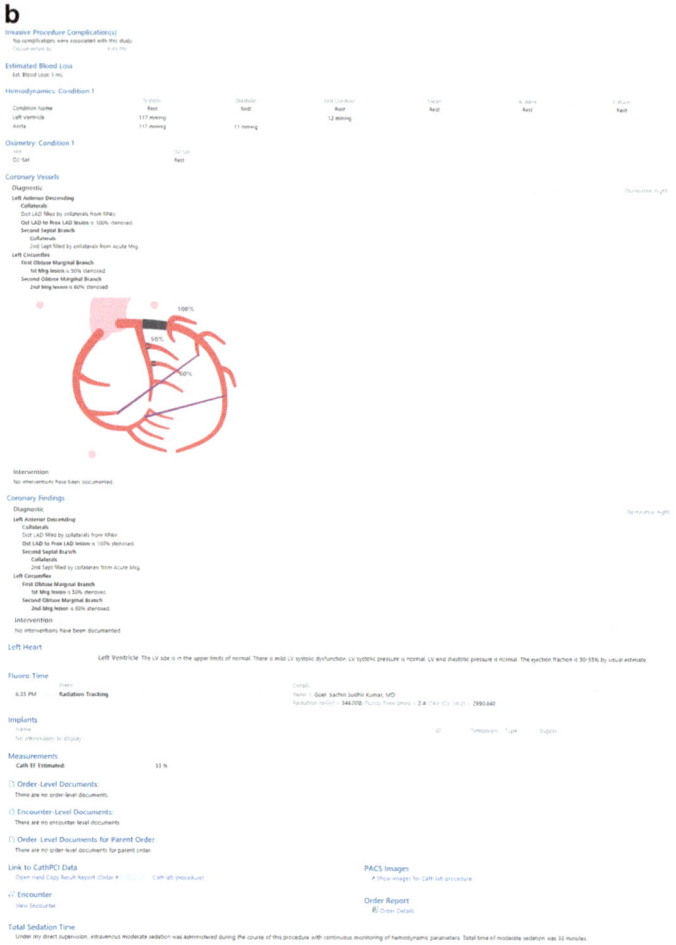

Fig. 7.3 (continued)

oped in 1975 with the use of a PDP 11 computer that took two and a half hours to determine the location of a single shot of radiation, but today it occurs in real time using desktop workstations [34]. An example of a MESR application is found in stereotactic radiosurgery with the Leksell GammaPlan® that is used to treat a variety of intracranial tumors and vascular disorders (Fig. 7.4) [35,

a

Fig. 7.4 (**a**) Leksell GammaPlan® report with tabular data describing the radiation treatment plan. (**b**) The GammaPlan® report includes annotated images indicating the prescription dose that will be used to treat a targeted brain metastasis (yellow isodose line). The green line indicates the 8 Gy isodose border to limit exposure to nontargeted tissues

b

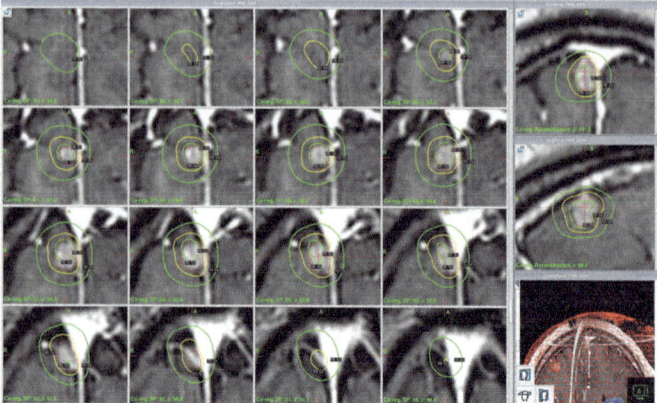

Fig. 7.4 (continued)

36]. In the future, the integration of radiation treatment plans with data from other MESR reports (e.g., diagnostic radiology and pathology) will be used to more effectively monitor long-term treatment efficacy as well as any potential adverse treatment effects.

7.2.4 Pathology

Surgical pathology has been a leader in synoptic reporting since the early 1990s [10, 37–39]. However, the incorporation of images into MESR reports has been slow to develop for a number of reasons, including the fact that the first whole slide imaging (WSI) system did not receive FDA clearance until 2017 [40]. Digital imaging in pathology faces several unique technical hurdles, including the need to define standards for image size and resolution, color models, image compression, and storage file types [41]. Whole slide imaging brings an added set of challenges as the storage needs increase substantially with each image being several gigabytes in size. Studies demonstrating diagnostic equivalence between the review of conventional glass slides and digital

WSI are encouraging, but workflow inefficiencies identified during the initial use of WSI viewing systems need to be addressed [42]. Novel concepts, including the use of gaming hardware, are being explored that could facilitate digital WSI analysis [43]. Standards developing organizations, including Digital Imaging and Communications in Medicine (DICOM) and the Integrating the Healthcare Enterprise (IHE), are actively engaged to address the unique imaging needs of pathology [44, 45]. After these technical hurdles are solved, the potential use of MESR in pathology should follow.

7.2.5 Dermatology

Dermatology is similar to gastroenterology in that it requires point-of-care imaging to document disease, but it is complicated by variable imaging methods (i.e., dedicated imaging systems versus consumer-grade cameras/smartphones), technical factors (i.e., lighting, angle, spatial resolution, magnification, color resolution), need for data encryption when transmitting images wirelessly, requirements for tagging images with patient information to match patient records, archival format (i.e., DICOM versus other image compression formats), and need for image annotation and accurate quantitative measurements [46]. Standards must be adopted to support interoperability with dermatologic images, including defining how the disease is classified (e.g., anatomical site, clinical impression, treatment plan) so that images may be correlated with pathology outcomes [47, 48]. The use of MESR in dermatology also faces privacy concerns as facial features, distinguishing tattoos, and unique body parts may inadvertently reveal a patient's identity. However, the potential for patients to use smartphones to document skin and other conditions in order to transmit images and video to healthcare providers is appealing, especially as telemedicine has become essential during the 2020 COVID-19 pandemic (Fig. 7.5). As in other fields, a DICOM workgroup is developing standards to address the technical challenges, but progress has been slow [49, 50].

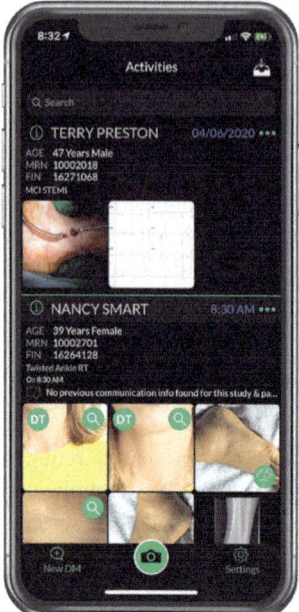 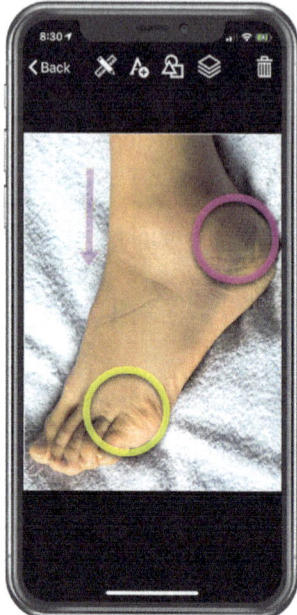

Fig. 7.5 Use of a smartphone camera to record patient images, which can be annotated to indicate sites of disease or injury (right), as well as allow for two-way communication between healthcare providers and patients. (Subject names are fictional. Images courtesy of Manabu Tokunaga, ZenSnapMD. com, Palo Alto, California, USA)

7.2.6   Radiology

Structured reporting in diagnostic radiology was first proposed a century ago, but the American College of Radiology finally declared at a 2016 Intersociety Summer Conference that "the era of unstructured radiology reports is coming to an end," and that structured data is required to support big data and machine learning initiatives [51]. Although structured reporting can exist without multimedia enhancement, Iyer reported in 2010 that the incorporation of representative images at the end of a text-based report can reduce the need for unnecessary consultations, increase confidence in treatment plans, and potentially alter patient management [52]. Nayak indicated in 2013 that referring physicians prefer image-embedded reports to improve comprehension of information contained in text-based reports [53]. Sadigh surveyed a group of clinicians in 2015 and found that 80% believed that MERR represents an improvement over text-only reports; furthermore, the surveyed physicians said that they would more likely refer patients to imaging facilities that offered MERR [54].

Several companies now offer commercially available MESR products. One example is Mint Medical GmbH (Heidelberg, Germany) with its mint Lesion™ software that is used for oncological screening, staging, and tumor response assessment (Figs. 7.6 and 7.7). The Mint Medical system supports many disease-specific applications (e.g., lung, colon, prostate, liver) and depicts radiological findings with elegant graphical formats that are easy for clinicians and patients to comprehend. The system also supports the calculation of several therapy response criteria, including RECIST 1.1, irRC, irRECIST, mRECIST, RANO, and others.

In 2010, Vining reentered the MESR field with a system called ViSion™ that works by recording key images and voice descriptions of findings, tagging the information with metadata linked to an ontology using natural language processing (NLP), and assembling an interactive multimedia report with related data from the EHR linked in timelines to show the evolution of disease (Fig. 7.8) [55]. The metadata that is used to tag each finding describes the anatomical location, radiological observation, and common data elements providing details about a particular diagnosis [56, 57]. ViSion overcomes an interoperability hurdle by recording screen images from any computer display, and it does not disrupt the radiologist's natural workflow of viewing and speaking about image findings since it uses NLP to produce structured data in the background. ViSion's comprehensive ontology relates multidisciplinary information from radiology, pathology, surgery, radiation therapy, and drug therapy in timelines from which medical outcomes can be calculated [58]. The interactive report is presented in a web browser, which allows for findings to be sorted and filtered, graphs to be displayed illustrating progression of disease, and external sources of additional information to be accessed via

a

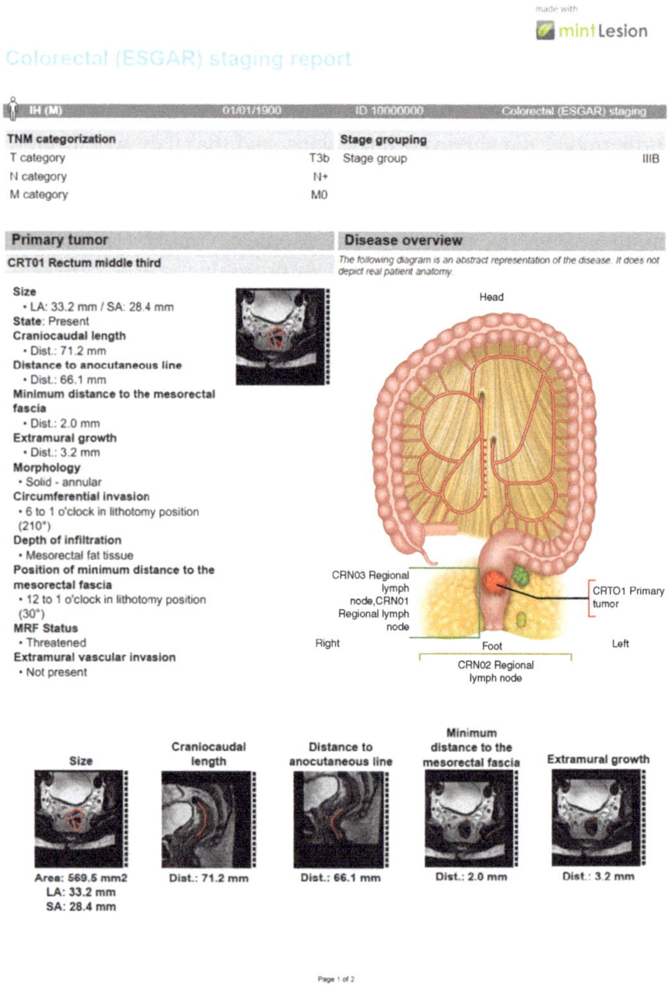

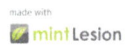

made with
mint Lesion

Colorectal (ESGAR) staging report

| IH (M) | 01/01/1900 | ID 10000000 | Colorectal (ESGAR) staging |

TNM categorization		Stage grouping	
T category	T3b	Stage group	IIIB
N category	N+		
M category	M0		

Primary tumor

CRT01 Rectum middle third

Size
• LA: 33.2 mm / SA: 28.4 mm
State: Present
Craniocaudal length
• Dist.: 71.2 mm
Distance to anocutaneous line
• Dist.: 66.1 mm
Minimum distance to the mesorectal fascia
• Dist.: 2.0 mm
Extramural growth
• Dist.: 3.2 mm
Morphology
• Solid - annular
Circumferential invasion
• 6 to 1 o'clock in lithotomy position (210°)
Depth of infiltration
• Mesorectal fat tissue
Position of minimum distance to the mesorectal fascia
• 12 to 1 o'clock in lithotomy position (30°)
MRF Status
• Threatened
Extramural vascular invasion
• Not present

Disease overview

The following diagram is an abstract representation of the disease. It does not depict real patient anatomy.

Head

CRN03 Regional lymph node, CRN01 Regional lymph node

CRT01 Primary tumor

Right · Foot · Left

CRN02 Regional lymph node

Size	Craniocaudal length	Distance to anocutaneous line	Minimum distance to the mesorectal fascia	Extramural growth
Area: 569.5 mm2 LA: 33.2 mm SA: 28.4 mm	Dist.: 71.2 mm	Dist.: 66.1 mm	Dist.: 2.0 mm	Dist.: 3.2 mm

Page 1 of 2

Fig. 7.6 (**a**) Mint Medical report for colorectal cancer staging with synoptic report findings on the left, graphical representation of disease on the right, and representative images below. (Courtesy of Mint Medical GMBH, Heidelberg, Germany). (**b**) Continuation of Mint Medical colorectal cancer staging report with additional key image recordings. (Courtesy of Mint Medical GMBH, Heidelberg, Germany)

b

Colorectal (ESGAR) staging report

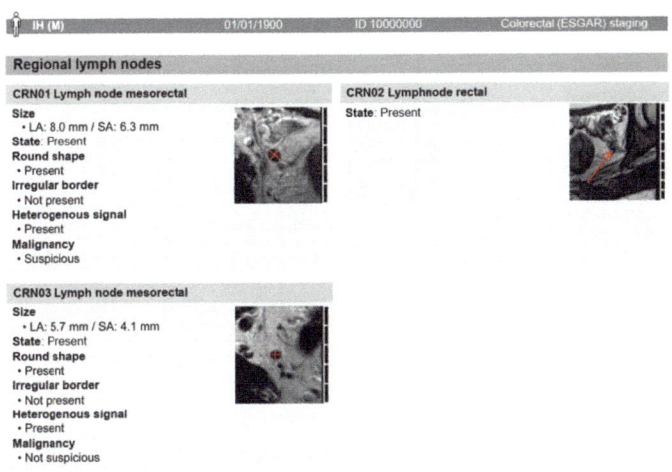

| IH (M) | 01/01/1900 | ID 10000000 | Colorectal (ESGAR) staging |

Regional lymph nodes

CRN01 Lymph node mesorectal

Size
• LA: 8.0 mm / SA: 6.3 mm
State: Present
Round shape
• Present
Irregular border
• Not present
Heterogenous signal
• Present
Malignancy
• Suspicious

CRN02 Lymphnode rectal

State: Present

CRN03 Lymph node mesorectal

Size
• LA: 5.7 mm / SA: 4.1 mm
State: Present
Round shape
• Present
Irregular border
• Not present
Heterogenous signal
• Present
Malignancy
• Not suspicious

Overall assessment

Peritoneum		Mesorectum	
Ascites	Absent	Tumor deposits	Present
Intestinal lumen width		Number of tumor deposits	3
Intestinal obstruction	Absent		

Fig. 7.6 (continued)

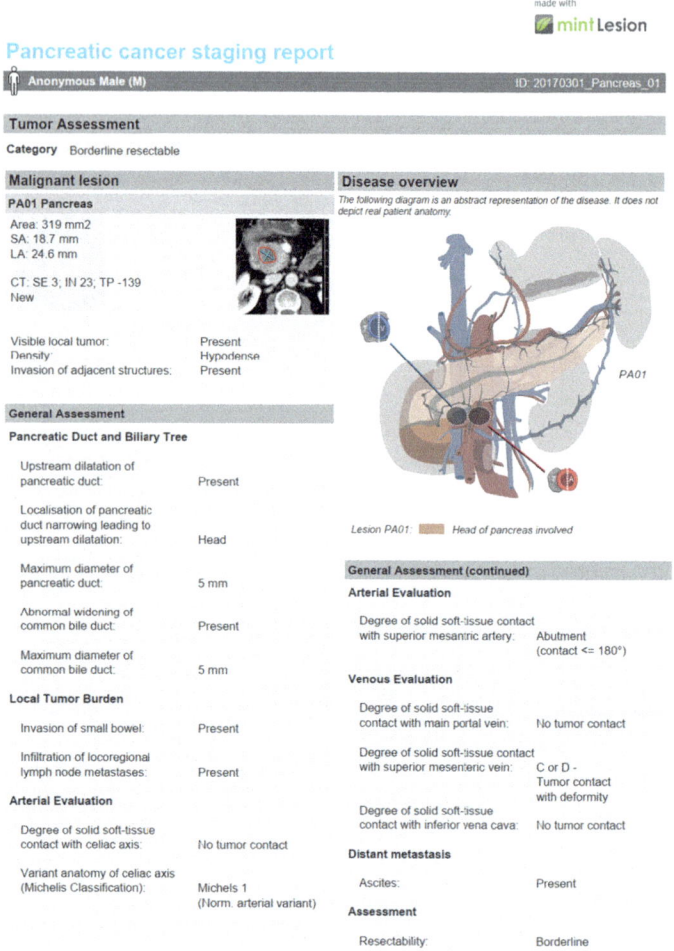

Fig. 7.7 Mint Medical report for pancreatic cancer staging with a key image in the top right, synoptic report on the left and bottom right, and graphical representation of disease in the upper right. (Courtesy of Mint Medical GMBH, Heidelberg, Germany)

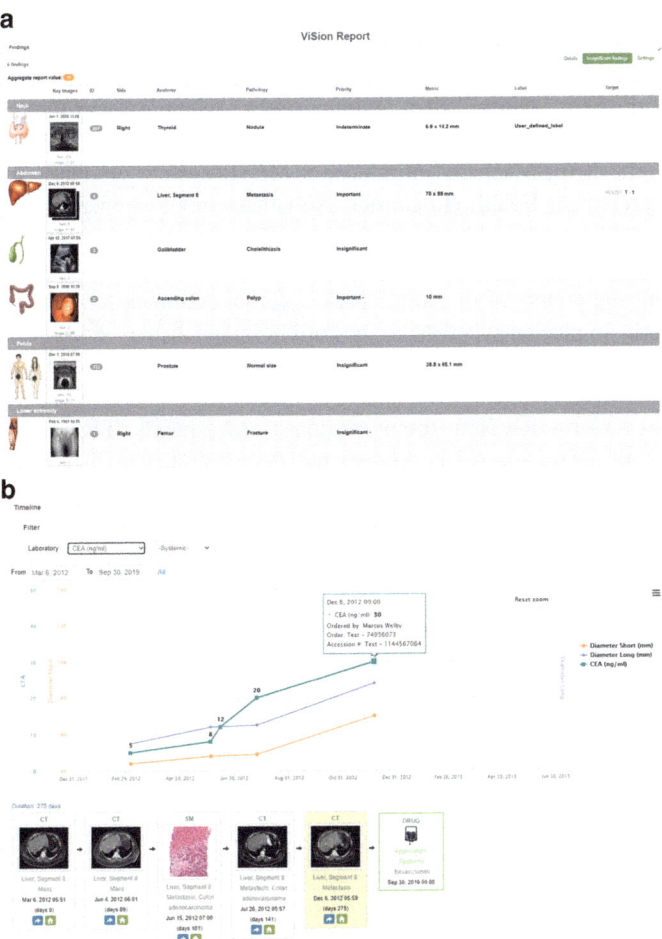

Fig. 7.8 (a) A ViSion™ composite report with the most recent image findings labeled with metadata to indicate anatomy, pathology (i.e., observation/diagnosis), metrics, and other elements. Hidden from view in this interactive report are the original text description and additional details (i.e., common data elements) associated with each finding, but those are available by clicking on each finding. (b) Clicking on the second finding in Fig. 7.10. A reveals more information, including a timeline illustrating the evolution of disease with images, graphed metrics, and related laboratory data. In this case, a patient with a liver mass is eventually biopsied and treated with monitoring of disease response

hyperlinks. The structured data that the system generates supports multiple advanced applications, including clinical trial management, translation of report elements to foreign languages, and actionable reporting (e.g., automatically assigning Lung-RADS designations to findings based on common data elements) [59].

In 2016, Machado introduced a MESR system produced by Carestream Health (Rochester, NY) that embeds hyperlinks to PACS images within dictated reports (Fig. 7.9) [60]. The system allows a radiologist to dictate a report in the usual manner but during the course of dictation speak a verbal command of "hyperlink" to place a hyperlink to the current image displayed in PACS within the text report. Image-related data (e.g., annotated measurements) are also automatically placed into a table that is used to perform RECIST tumor response assessments (Fig. 7.10). Early evaluation of the system has demonstrated high rates of acceptance, particularly among radiology trainees and for the

IMPRESSION:

1. Complex tear involving the posterior horn and body of the medial meniscus. Components include undersurface tear of the body (series 5, image 26) and free edge radial tear of the posterior horn (series 7, image 17).

2. Several small focal articular cartilage abnormalities, including among others a 6 mm high-grade inferior trochlear lesion (series 7, image 20) and fraying of the weightbearing medial femoral condyle cartilage adjacent to the meniscal tear.

3. Edema around the iliotibial band which can be seen in the clinical setting of iliotibial band syndrome.

4. Multilobulated intramuscular mass lesion with fluid-fluid levels within the vastus lateralis muscle thought likely to represent a vascular malformation/hemangioma. One of the larger components measures (4.8 cm x 2.5 cm) (series 8, image 32).

XXXXXX XXXX, M.D
Attending Musculoskeletal Radiologist

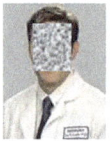

Final Sign Date/Time: 7/21/2021 4:50 PM

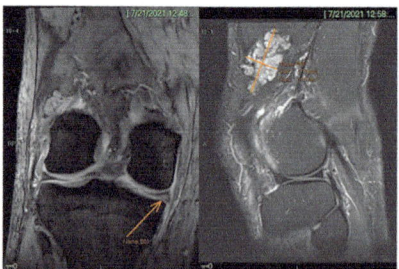

Fig. 7.9 Interactive multimedia report for an MRI examination of a knee illustrating a medial meniscus tear and an incidental vascular lesion. Note that hyperlinks corresponding to PACS images are embedded within the report impression. The report also contains copies of images illustrating the key findings (bottom right). (Courtesy of Dr. Cree Gaskin, UVA Health, Charlottesville, Virginia, USA)

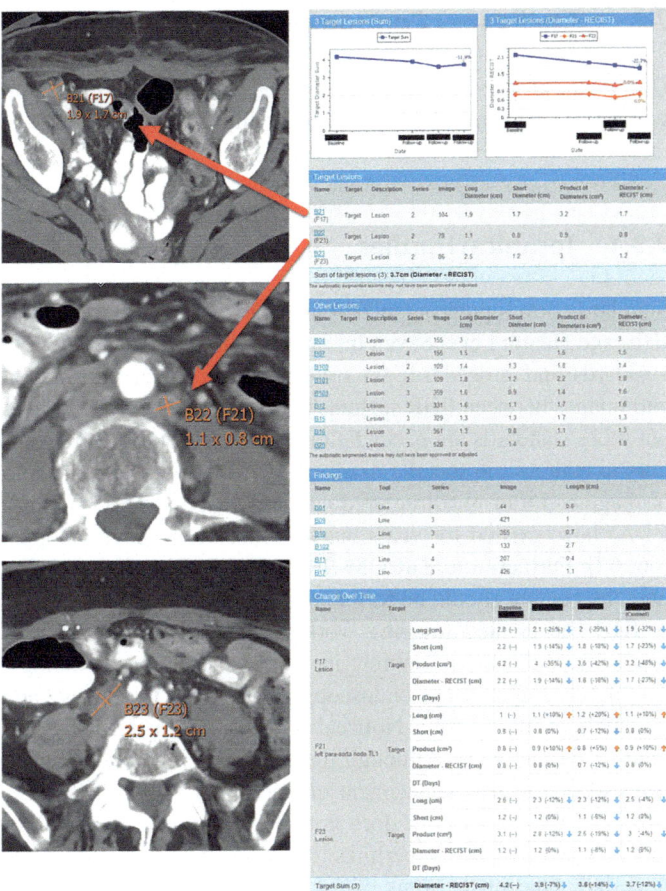

Fig. 7.10 MMICR report records image measurements into a table and auto-mates the calculation of RECIST disease response criteria. Hyperlinks in the table provide access to PACS images containing the corresponding measurements. (Courtesy of Dr. Les Folio, National Institutes of Health, Bethesda, Maryland, USA)

reporting of certain modalities, including computed tomography (CT), magnetic resonance imaging (MR), and positron emission tomography (PET) [61]. This interactive multimedia reporting solution was subsequently acquired by Royal Philips (Eindhoven, Netherlands) in 2019 [62].

7.3   Challenges Confronting Clinical Adoption

Despite the promise of MESR to advance medical communication, widespread clinical adoption has been hindered by a number of technical, human, and economic barriers.

7.3.1   Technical Hurdles

Standards developing organizations (SDOs), including DICOM, IHE, and Health Level Seven International (HL7), are developing standards and procedures for transmitting medical information and images between EHR systems to accomplish interoperability, but more standards are needed along with their adoption by vendors to address the specific needs of MESR [63–65]. Methods to package and transmit structured data (e.g., DICOM-SR and HL7 CDA) have existed for years but have not been widely adopted [66, 67]. Furthermore, DICOM-SR and HL7 CDA do not define how the content should be formulated or standardized.

IHE has created imaging workflows to address the unique needs of multiple specialties, including radiology, cardiology, dental, ophthalmology, endoscopy, pathology, pharmacy, and radiation oncology [68]. Noticeably absent from the list is the field of dermatology. Although the IHE has created a technical framework for the Management of Radiology Report Templates (MRRT), that framework does not address the specific requirements of MESR with hyperlinks to images and clinical information [69]. One of the aims of the HIMSS-SIIM IMR technical workgroup during the past couple of years has been to propose standards that will support the implementation of MESR.

In addition to defining MESR standards that will provide access to multimedia content (images, voice, text, lab, etc.), standards need to be created to allow for the distribution of interactive content among EHRs and patient portals. These types of standards are now being considered by various SDOs.

The National Cancer Institute (NCI) of the National Institutes of Health (NIH) has pursued its own set of interoperability standards through its Cancer Bioinformatics Grid (caBIG™) initiative that provides an infrastructure for generating and distributing research data, results, and tools using shared data standards and shared data models [70]. A product of caBIG™ has been the Annotated Image Markup (AIM) standard proposed in 2010 to support the capture and exchange of image measurements and other forms of image annotation between systems [71]. Although Rubin has demonstrated the utility of AIM, commercial adoption has been slow [72].

Multiple imaging and information exchange standards are continuing to be developed; consequently, harmonization of these standards will be required. Recent developments, including DICOMweb and HL7 FHIR, should facilitate interaction between imaging and EHR systems, respectively [73, 74]. The Substitutable Medical Applications, Reusable Technologies on Fast Healthcare Interoperability Resources (SMART on FHIR) initiative is an open, standards-based method for integrating third-party applications with EHR systems [75]. SMART on FHIR should overcome the technical hurdles that have plagued EHR systems since their inception by transforming them into platforms that can host innovative third-party MESR solutions that may not have been conceived previously by EHR vendors.

The development of a comprehensive medical ontology is needed to support MESR, particularly when relating and connecting disparate sources of information from the medical record. Although multiple ontologies exist that are used in EHR systems (e.g., CPT, ICD-10-CM, RxNorm, LOINC, SNOMED-CT, RadLex, etc.), each is missing domain-specific terminology and there is little interoperability between ontologies [76–81]. Harmonization of medical concepts and terminologies across disciplines remains a challenge.

Patient privacy and data security are additional technical hurdles that confront MESR implementation. MESR reports containing patient-identifying images (e.g., dermatology) present unique privacy concerns that require mitigation. In addition, the transmission of MESR reports containing hyperlinks between institutions needs to be addressed as hyperlinks may be perceived as a security risk in light of recent ransomware attacks targeting hospitals [82].

7.3.2 Human Impediments

Despite the appeal of MESR, multiple human factors impede its clinical acceptance. Structured reporting, and more specifically MESR, is perceived as being time-consuming, disrupting natural workflow, and producing less complete reports [83]. Others think that MESR adds little value, restricts freedom of expression, and creates legal liabilities, particularly when it produces a record of what may or may not have been reported using multimedia content [84]. Unfortunately, many referring physicians are also unaware of MESR's existence or potential benefits, thus contributing to a lack of demand.

Future studies need to demonstrate an improvement in MESR's communication efficiency, especially when considering the time that it takes for a clinician to assimilate information from siloed EHR systems. With the coming of artificial intelligence/machine learning (AI/ML) for automated disease detection, classification, and reporting, efficiency gains should be achieved to counter the perception that MESR is burdensome. In fact, given AI/ML's potential to report more sites of disease and in greater detail, MESR may become essential for effectively managing and presenting excessive amounts of data.

MESR has the potential to improve patient safety by connecting EHR data to reveal trends that may otherwise have gone unrecognized and to guide clinicians toward rendering more precise diagnoses, particularly when radiology–pathology correlation is achieved using MESR [85]. Innovative designs will overcome many of these human obstacles, and direct marketing of MESR's benefits to consumers may help to create public demand [86].

7.3.3 Economic Incentives

The lack of economic incentives has been an Achilles heel for MESR development. In 2018, EHR vendors began to open their proprietary systems and offer developer programs for interfacing third-party applications via application programming interfaces

(APIs), similar to the way that the smartphone industry has established a platform for hosting various applications [87]. However, similar to the smartphone industry, EHR vendors initially proposed taking up to 30% of gross revenues from application providers in exchange for hosting an application in the EHR ecosystem [88]. Pushback from third-party developers recently caused EHR vendors to restructure their pricing models [89].

Government policies have had a profound effect on the development and adoption of EHR systems. In the United States, the American Recovery and Reinvestment Act (ARRA) of 2009 incentivized the adoption of EHR systems [90]. The Health Information Technology for Economic and Clinical Health (HITECH) Act, part of the ARRA, subsequently established the Office of the National Coordinator for Health Information Technology (ONC), which continues to establish policies that are shaping the EHR landscape [91]. The Twenty-First Century Cures Act of 2015 led to the development of healthcare information exchanges and started efforts toward interoperability [92]. In July 2020, the Centers for Medicare and Medicaid Services (CMS) released its Interoperability and Patient Access (IPA) final rule, which requires the adoption of standards, including SMART on FHIR, to promote interoperability and allow for third-party access to patient data with proper clearance [93].

Undoubtedly, the greatest factor that will drive the adoption of MESR will be the transition from traditional fee-for-service reimbursement to pay-for-performance (i.e., value-based healthcare) [94]. As reimbursement is tied to increasing value, measuring outcomes, and improving clinician and patient experiences, MESR can play a pivotal role [95]. In the early stages of pay-for-performance in the United States, imaging-related quality metrics have been limited to simple measures, for example, determining what percentage of carotid imaging reports contain stenosis measurements [96]. However, as MESR continues to evolve and is capable of producing more connected and comprehensive patient analysis, the very use of MESR could become a quality metric in itself that will accelerate the adoption of MESR.

7.4   Conclusion

Communication worldwide is evolving as people embrace new forms of learning and information exchange; however, medical practices have been slow to adopt MESR reporting due to a number of technical, human, and economic factors. Vendors are now offering commercial MESR solutions, and EHR vendors have recently opened their systems to third-party innovation; thus, the future for MESR is promising. More work is required to achieve seamless interoperability between MESR and EHR systems, and industry groups such as the HIMSS-SIIM IMR workgroup are championing this effort. MESR will continue to evolve, and its role in value-based healthcare should drive its widespread adoption.

Conflicts of Interest VisionSR, Majority owner and CEO; Bracco Diagnostics, Royalties.

References

1. Folio LR, Machado LB, Dwyer AJ. Multimedia-enhanced radiology reports: concept, components, and challenges. Radiographics. 2018;38:462–82.
2. Moreno R, Mayer RE. Cognitive principles of multimedia learning: the role of modality and contiguity. J Educ Psychol. 1999;91:358–68.
3. Mayer RE. Applying the science of learning to medical education. Med Educ. 2010;44:543–9.
4. Yue C, et al. Applying the cognitive theory of multimedia learning: an analysis of medical animations. Med Educ. 2013;47:375–87.
5. Roth CJ, Clunie DA, Vining DJ, et al. Multispecialty enterprise imaging workgroup consensus on interactive multimedia reporting current state and road to the future: HIMSS-SIIM collaborative white paper. J Digit Imaging. 2021;34:495–522.
6. Ringeval M, et al. Fitbit-based interventions for healthy lifestyle outcomes: systematic review and meta-analysis. J Med Internet Res. 2020;22:e23954.
7. Eberhardt SC, Heilbrun ME. Radiology report value equation. Radiographics. 2018;38:1888–96.
8. Finny JM, Watson EJ. A report of cases illustrating the aid of the roentgen rays in the diagnosis of intrathoracic tumours. Br Med J. 1902;1:633–6.

9. Kaska SC, Weinstein JN. Ernest Amory Codman, 1869-1940: a pioneer of evidence-based medicine: the end result idea. Spine. 1998;23:629–33.
10. Markel SF, Hirsch SD. Synoptic surgical pathology reporting. Hum Pathol. 1991;22:807–10.
11. Hickey PM. Standardization of roentgen-ray reports. AJR. 1922;9:422–5.
12. Nelson TH. Complex information processing: a file structure for the complex, the changing and the indeterminate. ACM '65: Proceedings of the 1965 20th national conference. 1965. p. 84–100. https://doi.org/10.1145/800197.806036.
13. Chen CC, Hoffer PB, Swett HA. Hypermedia in radiology: computer-assisted education. J Digit Imaging. 1989;2:48–55.
14. Jaffe CC, Lynch PJ, Smeulders AW. Hypermedia techniques for diagnostic imaging instruction: videodisk echocardiography encyclopedia. Radiology. 1989;171:475–80.
15. Korein J, Kricheff II, Chase NE, Randt CT. Computer processing of neuroradiological reports. An introduction to the application of the variable-field-length format and MEDTRAN. Radiology. 1965;84:197–203.
16. Schramm C, Goldberg M, Pagurek B. Multimedia radiological reports: creation and playback. J Digit Imaging. 1989;2:106–13.
17. Goldberg M, et al. A multimedia medical communication link between a radiology department and an emergency department. J Digit Imaging. 1989;2:92–8.
18. Bellon E, et al. Multimedia e-mail systems for computer-assisted radiological communication. Med Inf. 1994;19:139–48.
19. Vining DJ, et al. REX: a rapid radiology reporting system. Radiology. 2000;217(Suppl P):698.
20. Brower RW, et al. The role of the personal computer in the cardiac catheterization laboratory: an integrated approach to information management. Comput Methods Prog Biomed. 1987;24:87–96.
21. Cheng DY, et al. MCAT—a multimedia cardiac angiogram tool. Proc Annu Symp Comput Appl Med Care. 1995:673–7.
22. Balogh N, et al. Cardiac digital image loops and multimedia reports over the internet using DICOM. Stud Health Technol Inform. 2002;90:148–51.
23. Olympus Advanced Reporting. https://medical.olympusamerica.com/technology/software-system-integration/electronic-medical-records/features-benefits/advanced-reporting. Accessed 3 Aug 2021.
24. EndoWorks® 7 Endoscopy Information Management Solution. https://medical.olympusamerica.com/technology/software-system-integration/endoscopy-support-software. Accessed 3 Aug 2021.
25. Lin OS, et al. Validation of colonoscopic findings from a structured endoscopic documentation database against manually collected medical records data. Surg Endosc. 2016;30:1607–13.
26. Douglas PS, et al. ACCF/ACR/AHA/ASE/ASNC/HRS/NASCI/RSNA/SAIP/SCAI/SCCT/SCMR 2008 Health Policy Statement on Structured Reporting in Cardiovascular Imaging. J Am Coll Cardiol. 2009;53:76–90.

27. Sanborn TA, et al. ACC/AHA/SCAI 2014 health policy statement on structured reporting for the cardiac catheterization laboratory: a report of the American College of Cardiology Clinical Quality Committee. Circulation. 2014;129:2578–609.
28. Mori Y, Igarashi T, Haraguchi R, Nakazawa K. A pen-based interface for generating graphical reports of findings in cardiac catheterization. Methods Inf Med. 2007;46:694–9.
29. Homorodean C, Olinic M, Olinic D. Development of a methodology for structured reporting of information in echocardiography. Med Ultrason. 2012;14:29–33.
30. Weintraub WS. Role of big data in cardiovascular research. J Am Heart Assoc. 2019;8:e012791.
31. GE Healthcare showcases new cardiovascular IT innovations. https://www.dicardiology.com/videos/video-ge-healthcare-showcases-new-cardiovascular-it-innovations. Accessed 3 Aug 2021.
32. Connected Cardiology begins here. Connect your cardiovascular enterprise with a single solution. https://www.youtube.com/watch?v=ms_QlXqk888. Accessed 3 Aug 2021.
33. Structured flexibility—with heart. https://www.siemens-healthineers.com/en-us/medical-imaging-it/cardiovascular-it-solutions/cardiovascular-imaging-information-solution. Accessed 3 Aug 2021.
34. Ganz JC. The development of dose planning. Prog Brain Res. 2014;215:111–6.
35. Guo F. 3-D treatment planning system-Leksell gamma knife treatment planning system. Med Dosim. 2018;43:177–83.
36. Leksell GammaPlan. Integrated treatment planning for gamma knife. https://www.elekta.com/radiosurgery/leksell-gammaplan. Accessed 3 Aug 2021.
37. Leslie KO, Rosai J. Standardization of the surgical pathology report: formats, templates, and synoptic reports. Semin Diagn Pathol. 1994;11:253–7.
38. Cancer protocol templates. https://www.cap.org/protocols-and-guidelines/cancer-reporting-tools/cancer-protocol-templates. Accessed 3 Aug 2021.
39. Nakhleh RE, et al. The future of College of American Pathologists cancer protocols: maintaining a commitment to patient safety while improving the user experience. Arch Pathol Lab Med. 2017;141:1153–4.
40. Food and Drug Administration, Office of the Commissioner: FDA allows marketing of first whole slide imaging system for digital pathology, 2017. http://www.fda.gov/news-events/press-announcements/fda-allows-marketing-first-whole-slide-imaging-system-digital-pathology. Accessed 3 Aug 2021.
41. Park S, Pantanowitz L. Digital imaging in pathology. Clin Lab Med. 2012;32:557–84.
42. Hanna MG, et al. Whole slide imaging equivalency and efficiency study: experience at a large academic center. Mod Pathol. 2019;32:916–28.

43. Yagi Y, et al. An ultra-high speed whole slide image viewing system. Anal Cell Pathol. 2012;35:65–73.
44. IHE Pathology and Laboratory Medicine (PaLM). https://wiki.ihe.net/index.php/Pathology_and_Laboratory_Medicine_(PaLM). Accessed 3 Aug 2021.
45. DICOM WG-26: Pathology. https://www.dicomstandard.org/activity/wgs/wg-26. Accessed 3 Aug 2021.
46. Quigley EA, et al. Technology and technique standards for camera-acquired digital dermatologic images—a systematic review. JAMA Dermatol. 2015;151:883–90.
47. Marghoob AA. Standards in dermatologic imaging. JAMA Dermatol. 2015;151:819–21.
48. Kenneweg KA, et al. Developing an international standard for the classification of surface anatomic location for use in clinical practice and epidemiologic research. J Am Acad Dermatol. 2019;80:1564–84.
49. DICOM WG-19: Dermatology. https://www.dicomstandard.org/activity/wgs/wg-19. Accessed 3 Aug 2021.
50. Caffery LJ, et al. Transforming dermatologic imaging for the digital era: metadata and standards. J Digit Imaging. 2018;31:568–77.
51. Kruskal JB, et al. Big data and machine learning-strategies for driving this bus: a summary of the 2016 Intersociety Summer Conference. J Am Coll Radiol. 2017;14:811–7.
52. Iyer VR, et al. Added value of selected images embedded into radiology reports to referring clinicians. J Am Coll Radiol. 2010;7:205–10.
53. Nayak L, et al. A picture is worth a thousand words: needs assessment for multimedia radiology reports in a large tertiary care medical center. Acad Radiol. 2013;20:1577–83.
54. Sadigh G, et al. Traditional text-only versus multimedia-enhanced radiology reporting: referring physicians' perceptions of value. J Am Coll Radiol. 2015;12:519–24.
55. Vining DJ, et al. A vision for radiology structured reporting. 97th Radiological Society of North America Proceedings (#LL-INS-WE7B), 11/2011. e-Pub.
56. Vining DJ, et al. Development of an ontological structure to relate signs/symptoms, pathology, radiological procedures, and treatments using anatomical locations as a common denominator. Poster presented at the meeting of the European Congress of Radiology, Vienna, Austria; 2019. https://doi.org/10.26044/ecr2019/C-2971.
57. Rubin DL, Kahn CE. Common data elements in radiology. Radiology. 2017;283:837–44.
58. Vining DJ, et al. Development of a multidisciplinary ontology for use in calculating medical outcomes. Poster presented at the meeting of the European Congress of Radiology, Vienna, Austria; 2020. https://doi.org/10.26044/ecr2020/C-11510

59. Vining DJ, et al. Use of common data elements and diagnostic templates in a clinical decision support system to produce higher-quality radiology reports. Poster presented at the meeting of the European Congress of Radiology, Vienna, Austria; 2020. https://doi.org/10.26044/ecr2020/C-14100

60. Machado LB, et al. Radiology reports with hyperlinks improve target lesion selection and measurement concordance in cancer trials. Am J Roentgenol. 2017;208:31–7.

61. Beesley SD, Patrie JT, Gaskin CM. Radiologist adoption of interactive multimedia reporting technology. J Am Coll Radiol. 2019;16:465–71.

62. Philips completes acquisition of Carestream Health's Healthcare Information Systems business in majority of relevant countries. https://www.philips.com/a-w/about/news/archive/standard/news/press/2019/20190801-philips-completes-acquisition-of-carestream-healths-healthcare-information-systems-business-in-majority-of-relevant-countries.html. Accessed 3 Aug 2021.

63. DICOM Digital Imaging and Communications in Medicine. https://www.dicomstandard.org. Accessed 3 Aug 2021.

64. IHE International—Integrating the Healthcare Enterprise. https://www.ihe.net. Accessed 3 Aug 2021.

65. HL7 International. https://www.hl7.org. Accessed 3 Aug 2021.

66. Noumeir R. Benefits of the DICOM structured report. J Digit Imaging. 2006;19:295–306.

67. HL7 International. CDA Release 2. https://www.hl7.org/implement/standards/product_brief.cfm?product_id=7. Accessed 3 Aug 2021.

68. IHE Domains. https://www.ihe.net/ihe_domains. Accessed 3 Aug 2021.

69. IHE Radiology Technical Framework Supplement—Management of Radiology Report Templates (MRRT). https://www.ihe.net/uploadedFiles/Documents/Radiology/IHE_RAD_Suppl_MRRT.pdf. Accessed 3 Aug 2021.

70. Harrington DP. Imaging and informatics at the National Cancer Institute, part 2. J Am Coll Radiol. 2006;3:169–70.

71. Channin DS, et al. The caBIG annotation and image markup project. J Digit Imaging. 2010;23:217–25.

72. Rubin DL, et al. ePAD: an image annotation and analysis platform for quantitative imaging. Tomography. 2019;5:170–83.

73. Khvastova M, et al. Towards Interoperability in Clinical Research—enabling FHIR on the open-source research platform XNAT. J Med Syst. 2020;44:137.

74. Vreeland A, et al. Considerations for exchanging and sharing medical images for improved collaboration and patient care: HIMSS-SIIM collaborative white paper. J Digit Imaging. 2016;29:547–58.

75. Mandel JC, et al. SMART on FHIR: a standards-based, interoperable apps platform for electronic health records. J Am Med Inform Assoc. 2016;23:899–908.

76. CPT® (Current Procedural Terminology). https://www.ama-assn.org/amaone/cpt-current-procedural-terminology. Accessed 3 Aug 2021.
77. International Classification of Diseases, Tenth Revision, Clinical Modification (ICD-10-CM). https://www.cdc.gov/nchs/icd/icd10cm.htm. Accessed 3 Aug 2021.
78. RxNorm. https://www.nlm.nih.gov/research/umls/rxnorm/index.html. Accessed 3 Aug 2021.
79. LOINC from Regenstrief. https://loinc.org. Accessed 3 Aug 2021.
80. SNOMED International. http://www.snomed.org. Accessed 3 Aug 2021.
81. RadLex radiology lexicon. https://www.rsna.org/en/practice-tools/data-tools-and-standards/radlex-radiology-lexicon. Accessed 3 Aug 2021.
82. Ransomware hits dozens of hospitals in an unprecedented wave. https://www.wired.com/story/ransomware-hospitals-ryuk-trickbot. Accessed 3 Aug 2021.
83. Johnson AJ, et al. Cohort study of structured reporting compared with conventional dictation. Radiology. 2009;253:74–80.
84. White WL, Stavola JM. The dark side of photomicrographs in pathology reports: liability and practical concerns hidden from view. J Am Acad Dermatol. 2006;54:353–6.
85. Filice RW. Radiology-pathology correlation to facilitate peer learning: an overview including recent artificial intelligence methods. J Am Coll Radiol. 2019;16(9 Pt B):1279–85.
86. Here's what innovators really need from EHR makers to move healthcare forward. https://www.healthcareitnews.com/news/heres-what-innovators-really-need-ehr-makers-move-healthcare-forward. Accessed 3 Aug 2021. ´
87. Sundvall E, et al. Graphical overview and navigation of electronic health records in a prototyping environment using Google earth and openEHR archetypes. Stud Health Technol Inform. 2007;129:1043–7.
88. App store fees, percentages, and payouts: what developers need to know. https://www.techrepublic.com/blog/software-engineer/app-store-fees-percentages-and-payouts-what-developers-need-to-know/#:~:text=For%20Android%20apps%2C%20developer%20fees,much%20less%20of%20an%20issue. Accessed 3 Aug 2021.
89. Epic App Orchard lowers participation fee for health IT developers. https://ehrintelligence.com/news/epic-app-orchard-lowers-participation-fee-for-health-it-developers. Accessed 3 Aug 2021.
90. Anumula N, Sanelli PC. Meaningful use. AJNR Am J Neuroradiol. 2012;33:1455–7.
91. The Office of the National Coordinator for Health Information Technology. https://www.healthit.gov. Accessed 3 Aug 2021.
92. Lye CT, et al. The 21st Century Cures Act and electronic health records one year later: will patients see the benefits? J Am Med Inform Assoc. 2018;25:1218–20.

93. CMS Interoperability and Patient Access final rule. https://www.cms.gov/Regulations-and-Guidance/Guidance/Interoperability/index. Accessed 3 Aug 2021.
94. Moser JW, et al. Pay for performance in radiology: ACR white paper. J Am Coll Radiol. 2006;3:650–64.
95. Heller RE 3rd. An analysis of quality measures in diagnostic radiology with suggestions for future advancement. J Am Coll Radiol. 2016;13:1182–7.
96. CMS.gov Centers for Medicare & Medicaid Services. CMS Measures Inventory. https://www.cms.gov/Medicare/Quality-Initiatives-Patient-Assessment-Instruments/QualityMeasures/CMS-Measures-Inventory. Accessed 3 Aug 2021.

Structured Reporting and Artificial Intelligence

8

Salvatore Claudio Fanni,
Michela Gabelloni,
Angel Alberich-Bayarri,
and Emanuele Neri

Contents

S. C. Fanni · M. Gabelloni · E. Neri
Academic Radiology, Department of Translational Research, University
of Pisa, Pisa, Italy

Italian Society of Medical and Interventional Radiology, SIRM
Foundation, Milan, Italy
e-mail: michela.gabelloni@unipi.it; emanuele.neri@unipi.it

A. Alberich-Bayarri (✉)
Quantitative Imaging Biomarkers in Medicine (QUIBIM SL), Valencia, Spain
e-mail: angel@quibim.com

© European Society of Medical Imaging Informatics
(EuSoMII) 2022
M. Fatehi, D. Pinto dos Santos (eds.), *Structured Reporting in
Radiology*, Imaging Informatics for Healthcare Professionals,
https://doi.org/10.1007/978-3-030-91349-6_8

8.1   Introduction

Structured radiology reporting has proved to be not only useful but also necessary in order to achieve completeness, comparability, and quantification and to minimize ambiguity [1]. The introduction of electronic medical record (EMR) holds the promise of advancing clinical research by allowing analysis of data contained in the radiology reports; unfortunately, this is extremely difficult in free-form text, while it is quicker and easier in structured reports [2].

Nowadays, structured reporting is still not widely used due to many reasons, such as the fact that technical difficulties and lack of integration make it time consuming; therefore, many radiology reports remain unstructured and use a free-form language [3].

Artificial intelligence (AI) may be the way to overcome these issues.

AI is a large area of study in the field of computer science, which deals with the development of tools able to perform human tasks or processes such as learning, reasoning, and self-correction [4].

A subfield of AI is natural language processing (NLP), also defined as "information extraction" or "text mining."

NLP is already part of our daily life, although little is known. For example, the system that separates valid e-mails from spam is based on text classification performed by an NLP tool.

NLP is a computer-based method that analyzes free-form text, in our case radiology reports, by combining linguistics, statistical, and AI methods, like machine learning (ML) or deep learning (DL).

The final output of this process is a structured format of specific itemized elements with a predefined organization and standardized terminology for each element [3].

From this analysis, NLP automatically identifies and extracts features, which ML or DL algorithm process, for example, to classify radiology reports [5].

Nevertheless, NLP will be useful in a transition period, passing from unstructured to structured reporting. The appropriateness of software and templates integration will allow for fast reporting also in a structured way [6–8], shortening the elapsed time in the reporting process [9]. The two biggest radiological scientific societies, the Radiological Society of North America (RSNA) and the European Society of Radiology (ESR), established the template library advisory panel (TLAP) to endorse specific structured reporting templates. The most relevant template database can be accessed through the RadReport portal (www.radreport.org), created by the RSNA.

The use of structured reporting templates is also the way in which images to be used for the creation of AI models can be properly annotated with the radiological findings.

A further step in the structured reporting is the inclusion of automatically generated quantitative imaging biomarkers in the report. The goal is not to create a fully quantitative report, which would resemble the way in which blood tests are reported, but to combine the findings detected by the radiologist with the associated annotations and quantitative metrics derived with a perfect combination between quantitative data and radiologist impressions.

8.2 Natural Language Processing: How Does It Work? An Overview on the Technical Workflow

8.2.1 Feature Extraction

NLP analysis starts off with preprocessing feature extraction, which is articulated in various steps. The different tools used in clinical practice and research implement in various ways the different possible steps that we are going to describe.

The first preprocessing steps are segmentation, sentence splitting, and tokenization.

Segmentation is defined as the identification of radiology reports sections, and the successive processing steps may be performed on every section or just a subset.

Further processing steps are divided into sentences, defined as sentence splitting, and into words, that is, tokenization [5].

Words, when separated, are characterized by considering the respective lexical root (stemming). Eventual spelling mistakes are fixed, and eventual abbreviations are expanded.

After normalization of the words, the syntactic analysis assigns part of speech of the words (noun, adjective, verb), their grammatical structure, and dependency relations [10].

The next stage is the semantic analysis, in order to identify for each word an individual concept and their modification by other contiguous terms. A concept is defined as a unique entity with a definite and unambiguous meaning. To standardize the medical language processing, the different software adopted medical lexicons. Lexicons are collections of precise definitions of concepts, each one with a preferred term and a list of possible synonymous or specific semantic [3]. Such lexicons are manually created by experts but may also be combined with existing lexicons; one of the most used is the Unified Medical Language System (UMLS) Metathesaurus [11].

When semantic analysis is completed, each individual concept is ideally output as a separate item in a structured format, which includes other contiguous concepts that modify it (e.g., for the concept of pneumonia, the anatomic location, or chronicity).

The primary NLP technologies used for these purposes are pattern matching and linguistic analysis.

Pattern matching is the simplest technique for searching text, and it is frequently integrated into more complex NLP tasks: it is based on matching of pattern, that is, a sequence of characters, to a given text.

Pattern matching, for example, is used in the above-mentioned process of stemming, in order to reduce a given word to its root and facilitate the connection to the relative lexicon concept.

Pattern matching could be used even to determine whether a concept is present or absent. NegEx is a pattern matching based on an algorithm, used to detect negation lexical words, such as "no" or "absent," within a small number of words before and after a specific concept [12].

Linguistic analysis is a more complex computer algorithm that uses syntactic and semantic knowledge to infer what concepts are cited in the text and how each concept is related to other contiguous concepts.

Limitations of this approach are ambiguity, incorrect grammar use, and misspellings.

An example of NLP resource based exclusively on linguistic analysis is Medical Extraction and Encoding (MedLEE), developed at New York Presbyterian Hospital [13]. MedLEE processes chest X-ray reports using semantic knowledge, and the final output is a structured format with a list of findings and associated modifiers for each finding [14].

8.2.2 Feature Processing, from Machine Learning to Deep Learning

The combined steps mentioned above produce the NLP features. Features are individual properties or characteristics of the subject of analysis. One of the simplest features in NLP is the *n*-grams, i.e., the consecutive number of words in a text.

However, concepts identified by semantic analysis have been shown to be more predictive features compared to *n*-grams [15]. Unfortunately, not all the words contained in the text can be reduced to a concept, such as conjunction or adverbs, however relevant and significant to achieve a complete comprehension of the radiological report.

The extracted features could be used to achieve text classification or information extraction. To solve this task, textual features can be processed by statistical, machine learning (ML), deep learning (DL) approach, or even hybrid approach.

ML is the branch of AI that studies the development of computer algorithms able to learn from data [16]. While the statistical approach utilizes hand-crafted statistics rules, the machine learning approach automatically generates the classification rules.

ML can be used even to achieve linguistic tasks.

The Statistical Assertion Classifier (StAC) performs the same function of the previously mentioned pattern-matching-based tool NegEx. However, StAC works with a completely different and more complex technique. In fact, StAC is an ML algorithm that learns what negations are by analyzing radiology reports previously labeled by humans for the presence/absence of negations [17].

The ML algorithm is mostly integrated in NLP processing with the purpose of classification of radiology reports analyzing the extracted features.

The simplest way is to classify reports by analyzing the presence/absence of findings and their possible combination.

For example, if findings such as pneumonia or infiltrates are described in a chest x-ray report by an NLP tool, then the report is likely classified as positive for pneumonia [18].

Machine learning algorithms perform report classification tasks by analyzing data and automatically determining which features correlate with a positive or negative result.

In order to achieve these results, machine learning methods previously require training labeled data to establish a connection between the extracted features and predefined class. Care must be taken in the choice of the number and type of data because the performance of the classifier strongly depends on the training set [19].

A subfield of machine learning is deep learning (DL). In DL, the algorithm learns without any prior human feature selection [20].

DL models are based on artificial neural networks (ANNs), inspired by the neural cortex, where each neuron is connected with other neurons [20].

ANNs are a collection of artificial neurons organized in multiple layers, structured as input, hidden computation, and output layers [21].

The information is fed through the input layer, processed through the hidden layers, and the result is produced from the output layer.

The most used ANNs are convolutional neural networks (CNNs) and recurrent neural networks (RNNs). A CNN model is usually composed of numerous convolutional layers followed by a few fully connected layers [22]. CNN uses a repeating pattern in the dataset [20].

As in images, repeating patterns also appear in the free-form text [23].

Conversely, RNNs process sequential information, which is ideal in NLP, because sentences are sequences of words. The neurons in RNNs are connected sequentially, like a long chain, each passing the respective output to the next neuron. The sequential passing of information creates a memory; unfortunately, in long-distance sentences, the "memory effect" loses effectiveness, while the memory diminishes passing through numerous layers.

To overcome this issue, a subtype of RNNs has been developed, the long short-term memory network, which is more effective for analyzing long and complex radiology reports [24].

DL algorithms have outperformed traditional NLP methods in various tasks, leading to a significant increase in research in this field [25].

For these reasons, it is expected that DL applications in NLP will play a largest and important role in clinical practice in coming years.

8.3   Application of Natural Language Processing in Radiology

NLP in radiology is already used for many purposes, and the largest application categories are the following:

– Identifying/classifying findings
– Identifying cases/cohort for research studies
– Identifying follow-up recommendations
– Imaging protocol determinations
– Diagnostic surveillance
– Assessing the quality of radiologic practice

The major benefit is automation and evaluation of large amounts of data in a reasonable time, while performing these tasks without using NLP and AI is at least unthinkable.

One of the first applications of NLP was **identifying/classifying findings**. In 1998, Knirsch et al. compared MedLEE, a traditional NLP tool based on linguistic analysis, with experts review in order to identify chest x-ray reports suspicious for tuberculosis. The purpose was to identify automatically from the radiological report of the patient who needs respiratory isolation protocol. The agreement was 89–92% focusing on the presence/absence of six pre-selected keywords in the report [26].

MedLEE is also one of the first NLP tools used for **identifying cases/cohort for research studies.**

Hripcsak et al. used MedLEE for large-scale research on radiological reports, in order to test four different hypotheses. The automated analysis has made it possible to analyze a huge number of reports: 889.921! [27].

AI represented one of the most important innovations in the NLP field; in fact, ML and DL methods outperformed different times the traditional tools. In order to compare different NLP tools, different quantitative parameters have been used. F1 score is one of these parameters; it is a harmonized average of sensitivity and positive predictive value (PPV) and is frequently used as an overall measure of NLP tools' performance.

An application of NLP has been to classify radiology reports of contrast material-enhanced CT of the chest performed to evaluate pulmonary embolism. In 2012, Chapman et al. developed an NLP tool named PeFinder (i.e., pulmonary embolism finder) for this purpose. PeFinder classified reports based on the presence/absence and location of pulmonary embolism, chronicity, and certainty. PeFinder applied an extension of NegEx to identify lexical clues and define concepts (i.e., pulmonary embolism). This simple technology achieved good results, such as high sensitivity and specificity [28].

Cheng et al. in 2018 compared a CNN model with peFinder, which was considered the best available software for this specific purpose.

However, the CNN model outperformed PeFinder based on F1 score (0.938 vs. 0.867) [29].

Miao et al. evaluated the extraction of BI-RADS findings from breast ultrasound reports. They compared three different types of NLP approach: a traditional role-based approach, a machine-learning approach, and an RNN model. The RNN model performed better than the other methods [30].

Another important application for NLP is the **automatic identification of follow-up recommendations** from radiology reports. Nowadays, this task remains challenging due to a lack of standardized/structured reporting.

In 2019, Carrodeguas et al. assessed about 1000 radiology reports for this purpose, evaluating traditional NLP tools (iSCOUT) and ML (Support Vector Machine) and DL models (RNN network). The highest F1 sore was achieved by ML models (0.85), while iSCOUT and DL models performed at 0.71.

Imaging protocol determination is a helpful application for NLP in radiology in order to save time and potentially standardize and decrease errors of contrast material injection.

In 2017, Trivedi et al. used the Watson DL protocol to evaluate the need for intravenous contrast injection in musculoskeletal MRI based on the free-text of clinical indication provided for the study. The DL protocol achieved an accepting accuracy (80–90%), resulting in a good clinical decision support tool [31].

Another important NLP task that needs to be mentioned is **diagnostic surveillance** in order to safeguard clinical practice and potentially reduce the chance of errors in communication between radiologists and clinicians. NLP tools developed for this specific task raise alerts for the presence of predetermined findings/conditions contained in the radiology report.

Rink et al. developed a hybrid approach involving a customized lexicon, manually defined patterns and an ML model (support vector machine) able to identify appendicitis based on individual statements of radiological reports. The model achieves a sensitivity of 91% and PPV of 83% [32].

Last but not least, NLP is a helpful tool for **quality assessment of radiologic practice**. NLP tools covering this task identify specific quality indicators used for internal quality assurance, comparison to guidelines, and legal purpose.

For example, Lacson et al. used iSCOUT to select reports with pulmonary nodules and verify the concordance between node management and recommendations from the Fleischner Society Guidelines [33].

8.4   Structured Reporting as AI Annotation Strategy

Appropriate implementation of structured reporting is based on templates. Integrating the healthcare enterprise (IHE) initiative developed a standard for the presentation of structured reports through the working group on Management of Radiology Reporting Templates (MRRT). It specifies which technology should be used for template development and describes how these templates should be managed and integrated into radiology information systems or PACS reporting orchestrators and their migration to these environments. In contrast, MRRT does not define how template-based reports are transmitted from a radiology information system or PACS to an electronic health record system.

Structured reports can also be stored in DICOM format since the current standard definition considers the "DICOM-SR" modality. In the standard, the guidelines to be followed in the DICOM-SR object creation and the encoding of the information contained are specified. Furthermore, DICOM-SR objects can also include the annotations (i.e., measurements, regions of interest, among others) performed by the radiologist using the tools available in a PACS workstation. Measurements and annotations provide meaningful information to complement the qualitative findings included in the report.

The combination of the HL7 standard with DICOM-SR enriches the report with clinical information relevant to patient diagnosis through the images obtained.

Structured reporting enables the development of deep learning algorithms thanks to the seamless annotation performed while reporting. Annotation is mainly performed today from retrospective data by NLP techniques, as seen in previous sections. Nevertheless, a risk to generate inaccuracies and uncertainties not only in annotation but also in the creation of deep learning models has already been in the case of the CheXNet paper [34, 35].

As an improved and scalable annotating methodology, research experiences have already demonstrated the feasibility of using the data from structured reports completed in clinical routine for training deep learning algorithms, highlighting the potential of structured reporting for the future of radiology in the context of AI and deep learning as the main technique applied [36–38].

8.5   Quantitative Structured Reporting

Structured reports can also be the way in which AI algorithms and image analysis results are communicated and integrated into hospital information systems such as the PACS, RIS, or EHR.

Quantitative features are today being generated in the form of imaging biomarkers by applying computational algorithms to the analysis of medical images. Computational imaging algorithms can either be based on AI (driven by data) or on conventional computer vision algorithms (driven by model). The main aim of quantitative imaging biomarkers is to early detect disease before symptoms, to establish a diagnosis and staging if the disease and symptoms are already present, to predict patient outcomes, and to evaluate treatment response during follow-up.

The extracted imaging biomarkers provide quantitative information on their spatial distribution (parametric images) and their magnitude (intensity). The textural analysis of signal intensity properties from different voxels in a region of interest, through the extraction of quantitative features, allows for the evaluation of first-order histogram characteristics (intensity, skewness, kurtosis) and second-order parameters (energy, information, correlation, among many others). The process of extracting hundreds or thousands of these features and using AI-based classifiers whose output is a clinical endpoint is called radiomics.

With regard to radiological workflow integration, even if these imaging biomarkers and radiomics capabilities may be available in a research or academic domain, their integration within radiology information systems such as the RIS and PACS is still not straightforward. As an example, we can obtain the percentage of the affected lung in the computed tomography images of a COVID-19 patient, but current systems will not allow integrating this value seamlessly in the radiology report (without manually typing it) or performing population-based queries such as "show me all cases analyzed during the last year with a % of affected lung higher than 20%."

The final results of AI and imaging biomarker extraction algorithms must be available in the radiology structured reporting environment in order for the radiologists to be able to accept, amend, or reject this information.

As of now, quantitative structured reports can be generated in a parallel streamline that allows integrating final reports as an annex to the conventional radiology reporting. These quantitative reports can be generated by the use of HTML or Jade templates that are installed in an environment or ecosystem hosting different applications and orchestrating AI analysis in the radiology routine. An example of the quantitative structured report obtained from the application of convolutional neural networks (CNNs) for the detection of ground glass opacities and the quantification of lung damage can be appreciated in Fig. 8.1.

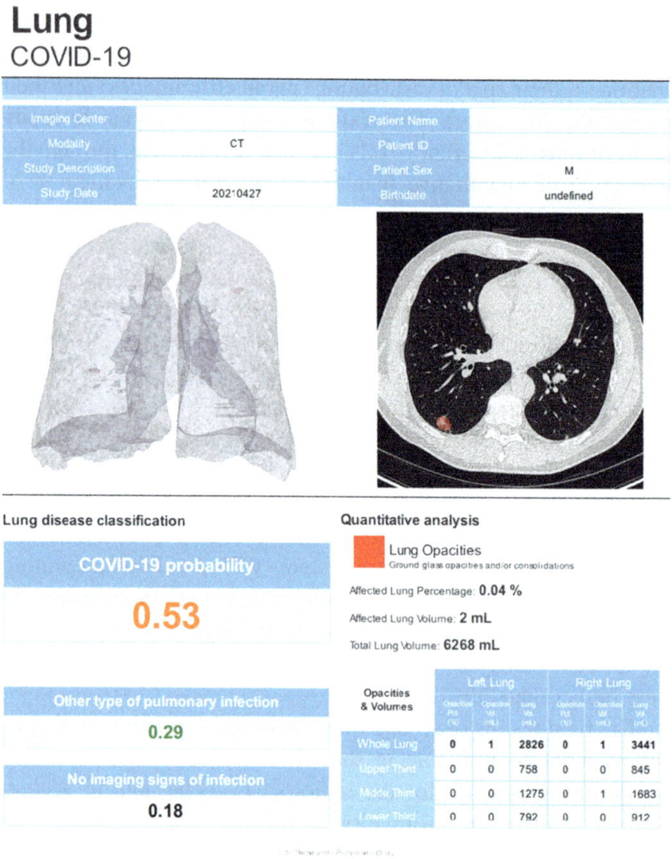

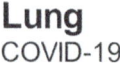

Lung
COVID-19

Imaging Center		Patient Name	
Modality	CT	Patient ID	
Study Description		Patient Sex	M
Study Date	2021 0427	Birthdate	undefined

Lung disease classification

COVID-19 probability

0.53

Other type of pulmonary infection

0.29

No imaging signs of infection

0.18

Quantitative analysis

Lung Opacities
Ground glass opacities and/or consolidations

Affected Lung Percentage: **0.04 %**

Affected Lung Volume: **2 mL**

Total Lung Volume: **6268 mL**

Opacities & Volumes	Left Lung			Right Lung		
	Opacities Pct (%)	Opacities Vol (mL)	Lung Vol (mL)	Opacities Pct (%)	Opacities Vol (mL)	Lung Vol (mL)
Whole Lung	0	1	2826	0	1	3441
Upper Third	0	0	758	0	0	845
Middle Third	0	0	1275	0	1	1683
Lower Third	0	0	792	0	0	912

Fig. 8.1 Quantitative structured report generated from an AI pipeline that calculates the percentage of the affected lung by COVID-19 opacities and the probability of being a positive case

References

1. European Society of Radiology (ESR). ESR paper on structured reporting in radiology. Insights. Imaging. 2018;9(1):1–7. https://doi.org/10.1007/s13244-017-0588-8. Epub 2018 Feb 19.
2. Institute of Medicine (US) Committee on Data Standards for Patient Safety. Key Capabilities of an Electronic Health Record System: Letter Report. Washington, DC: National Academies Press (US); 2003. https://www.ncbi.nlm.nih.gov/books/NBK221802/.
3. Cai T, Giannopoulos AA, Yu S, Kelil T, Ripley B, Kumamaru KK, Rybicki FJ, Mitsouras D. Natural language processing technologies in radiology research and clinical applications. Radiographics. 2016;36(1):176–91. https://doi.org/10.1148/rg.2016150080.
4. Kok JN, Boers EJW, Kosters WA, van der Putten P, Poel M. Artificial intelligence: definition, trends, techniques and cases. Encyclopedia of Life Support Systems (EOLSS). UNESCO-EOLSS.
5. Pons E, Braun LM, Hunink MG, Kors JA. Natural language processing in radiology: a systematic review. Radiology. 2016;279(2):329–43. https://doi.org/10.1148/radiol.16142770.
6. Martí-Bonmatí L, Ruiz-Martínez E, Ten A, Alberich-Bayarri A. How to integrate quantitative information into imaging reports for oncologic patients. Radiologia. 2018;60(Suppl 1):43–52. https://doi.org/10.1016/j.rx.2018.02.005. Epub 2018 Mar 28.
7. Montoliu-Fornas G, Martí-Bonmatí L. Magnetic resonance imaging structured reporting in infertility. Fertil Steril. 2016;105(6):1421–31. https://doi.org/10.1016/j.fertnstert.2016.04.005. Epub 2016 Apr 19.
8. Medina García R, Torres Serrano E, Segrelles Quilis JD, Blanquer Espert I, Martí Bonmatí L, Almenar Cubells D. A systematic approach for using DICOM structured reports in clinical processes: focus on breast cancer. J Digit Imaging. 2015;28(2):132–45. https://doi.org/10.1007/s10278-014-9728-6.
9. Segrelles JD, Medina R, Blanquer I, Martí-Bonmatí L. Increasing the efficiency on producing radiology reports for breast cancer diagnosis by means of structured reports. A comparative study. Methods Inf Med. 2017;56(3):248–60. https://doi.org/10.3414/ME16-01-0091. Epub 2017 Feb 21.
10. Kao A, Poteet S. Overview. In: Kao A, Poteet S, editors. Natural language processing and text mining. New York, NY: Springer; 2007. p. 1–7.
11. National Library of Medicine (U.S.). UMLS reference Manual, Chapter 1, Introduction to the UMLS. 2009. http://www.ncbi.nlm.nih.gov/books/NBK9675/. Accessed 20 Mar 2021.
12. Chapman WW, Bridewell W, Hanbury P, Cooper GF, Buchanan BG. A simple algorithm for identifying negated findings and diseases in discharge summaries. J Biomed Inform. 2001;34(5):301–10.

13. Friedman C, Alderson PO, Austin JH, Cimino JJ, Johnson SB. A general natural-language text processor for clinical radiology. J Am Med Inform Assoc. 1994;1(2):161–74.

14. Friedman C, Shagina L, Lussier Y, Hripcsak G. Automated encoding of clinical documents based on natural language processing. J Am Med Inform Assoc. 2004;11(5):392–402.

15. Yu S, Kumamaru KK, George E, et al. Classification of CT pulmonary angiography reports by presence, chronicity, and location of pulmonary embolism with natural language processing. J Biomed Inform. 2014;52:386–93.

16. Goecks J, Jalili V, Heiser LM, Gray JW. How machine learning will transform biomedicine. Cell. 2020;181(1):92–101. https://doi.org/10.1016/j.cell.2020.03.022.

17. Uzuner O, Zhang X, Sibanda T. Machine learning and rule-based approaches to assertion classification. J Am Med Inform Assoc. 2009;16(1):109–15.

18. Elkin PL, Froehling D, Wahner-Roedler D, et al. NLP-based identification of pneumonia cases from free-text radiological reports. AMIA Annu Symp Proc. 2008;2008:172–6.

19. Cheng LT, Zheng J, Savova GK, Erickson BJ. Discerning tumor status from unstructured MRI reports—completeness of information in existing reports and utility of automated natural language processing. J Digit Imaging. 2010;23(2):119–32. https://doi.org/10.1007/s10278-009-9215-7. Epub 2009 May 30.

20. Soffer S, Ben-Cohen A, Shimon O, Amitai MM, Greenspan H, Klang E. Convolutional neural networks for radiologic images: a radiologist's guide. Radiology. 2019;290:590–606.

21. Chartrand G, Cheng PM, Vorontsov E, et al. Deep learning: a primer for radiologists. Radiographics. 2017;37:2113–31.

22. Khaki S, Wang L, Archontoulis SV. A CNN-RNN framework for crop yield prediction. Front Plant Sci. 2020;10:1750. https://doi.org/10.3389/fpls.2019.01750.

23. Kim Y. Convolutional neural networks for sentence classification. arXiv preprint arXiv:14085882. 2014. https://arxiv.org/abs/1408.5882. Accessed Mar 2021.

24. Hochreiter S, Schmidhuber J. Long short-term memory. Neural Comput. 1997;9:1735–80.

25. Ruder S. NLP's ImageNet moment has arrived. 2018. https://thegradient.pub/nlp-imagenet/. Accessed Mar 2021.

26. Knirsch CA, Jain NL, Pablos-Mendez A, Friedman C, Hripcsak G. Respiratory isolation of tuberculosis patients using clinical guidelines and an automated clinical decision support system. Infect Control Hosp Epidemiol. 1998;19(2):94–100.

27. Hripcsak G, Austin JH, Alderson PO, Friedman C. Use of natural language processing to translate clinical information from a database of 889,921 chest radiographic reports. Radiology. 2002;224(1):157–63.

28. Chapman BE, Lee S, Kang HP, Chapman WW. Document-level classification of CT pulmonary angiography reports based on an extension of the ConText algorithm. J Biomed Inform. 2011;44(5):728–37. https://doi.org/10.1016/j.jbi.2011.03.011. Epub 2011 Apr 1.

29. Chen MC, Ball RL, Yang L, et al. Deep learning to classify radiology free-text reports. Radiology. 2018;286:845–52.

30. Miao S, Xu T, Wu Y, Xie H, Wang J, Jing S, Zhang Y, Zhang X, Yang Y, Zhang X, Shan T, Wang L, Xu H, Wang S, Liu Y. Extraction of BI-RADS findings from breast ultrasound reports in Chinese using deep learning approaches. Int J Med Inform. 2018;119:17–21. https://doi.org/10.1016/j.ijmedinf.2018.08.009. Epub 2018 Aug 18.

31. Trivedi H, Mesterhazy J, Laguna B, Vu T, Sohn JH. Automatic determination of the need for intravenous contrast in musculoskeletal MRI examinations using IBM Watson's natural language processing algorithm. J Digit Imaging. 2018;31:245–51.

32. Rink B, Roberts K, Harabagiu S, et al. Extracting actionable findings of appendicitis from radiology reports using natural language processing. AMIA Jt Summits Transl Sci Proc. 2013;2013:221.

33. Lacson R, Prevedello LM, Andriole KP, et al. Factors associated with radiologists' adherence to Fleischner Society guidelines for management of pulmonary nodules. J Am Coll Radiol. 2012;9(7):468–73.

34. Rajpurkar P, Irvin J, Zhu K et al. CheXNet: radiologist-level pneumonia detection on chest X-rays with deep learning. 2017. http://arxiv.org/abs/1711.05225v3. Accessed 30 Mar 2021.

35. Oakden-Rayner L. CheXNet: an in-depth review. 2018. https://lukeoakdenrayner.wordpress.com/2018/01/24/chexnet-an-in-depth-review/. Accessed 30 Mar 2021.

36. Pinto dos Santos D. The value of structured reporting for AI: opportunities, applications and risks. 2019. https://doi.org/10.1007/978-3-319-94878-2_7.

37. Bizzo BC, Almeida RR, Alkasab TK. Computer-assisted reporting and decision support in standardized radiology reporting for cancer imaging. JCO Clin Cancer Inform. 2021;5:426–34. https://doi.org/10.1200/CCI.20.00129.

38. Goldberg-Stein S, Chernyak V. Adding value in radiology reporting. J Am Coll Radiol. 2019;16(9 Pt B):1292–8. https://doi.org/10.1016/j.jacr.2019.05.042.

GPSR Compliance

The European Union's (EU) General Product Safety Regulation (GPSR) is a set of rules that requires consumer products to be safe and our obligations to ensure this.

If you have any concerns about our products, you can contact us on ProductSafety@springernature.com

In case Publisher is established outside the EU, the EU authorized representative is:

Springer Nature Customer Service Center GmbH
Europaplatz 3
69115 Heidelberg, Germany

Batch number: 10100290

Printed by Printforce, the Netherlands